BIOMECHANICAL EVALUATION OF MOVEMENT IN SPORT AND EXERCISE

Biomechanical Evaluation of Movement in Sport and Exercise offers a comprehensive and practical sourcebook for students, researchers and practitioners involved in the quantitative evaluation of human movement in sport and exercise.

This unique text sets out the key theories underlying biomechanical evaluation, and explores the wide range of biomechanics laboratory equipment and software that is now available. Advice concerning the most appropriate selection of equipment for different types of analysis, as well as how to use the equipment most effectively, is also offered.

The book includes coverage of:

- Measurement in the laboratory and in the field
- Motion analysis using video and on-line systems
- Measurement of force and pressure
- Measurement of muscle strength using isokinetic dynamometry
- Electromyography
- Computer simulation and modelling of human movement
- Data processing and data smoothing
- Research methodologies

Written and compiled by subject specialists, this authoritative resource provides practical guidelines for students, academics and those providing scientific support services in sport science and the exercise and health sciences.

Carl J. Payton is Senior Lecturer in Biomechanics at Manchester Metropolitan University, UK. **Roger M. Bartlett** is Professor of Sports Biomechanics in the School of Physical Education, University of Otago, New Zealand.

BIOMECHANICAL EVALUATION OF MOVEMENT IN SPORT AND EXERCISE

The British Association of Sport and
Exercise Sciences Guidelines

Edited by Carl J. Payton and Roger M. Bartlett

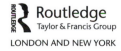

Routledge
Taylor & Francis Group

LONDON AND NEW YORK

First published 2008
by Routledge
2 Park Square, Milton Park, Abingdon, Oxon OX14 4RN

Simultaneously published in the USA and Canada
by Routledge
270 Madison Ave, New York, NY 10016

Routledge is an imprint of the Taylor & Francis Group, an informa business

Typeset in Sabon by Keyword Group Ltd
Printed and bound in Great Britain by TJ International Ltd,
Padstow, Cornwall

British Library Cataloguing-in-Publication Data
A catalogue record for this book is available from the British Library

Library of Congress Cataloging in Publication Data
Biomechanical evaluation of movement in sport and exercise: the British
Association of Sport and Exercise Science guide / edited by Carl Payton and
Roger Bartlett.
p. ; cm.
Includes bibliographical references.
ISBN 978-0-415-43468-3 (hardcover) – ISBN 978-0-415-43469-0 (softcover)
1. Human mechanics. 2. Exercise–Biomechanical aspects.
3. Sports–Biomechanical aspects. I. Payton, Carl. II. Bartlett, Roger.
III. British Association of Sport and Exercise Sciences.

[DNLM: 1. Movement–physiology. 2. Biometry–methods.
3. Exercise–physiology. 4. Models, Statistical. WE 103 B6139 2007]
QP303.B557 2007 *2008*
612.7′6–dc22   2007020521
ISBN10: 0-415-43468-8 (hbk)
ISBN10: 0-415-43469-6 (pbk)
ISBN10: 0-203-93575-6 (ebk)

ISBN13: 978-0-415-43468-3 (hbk)
ISBN13: 978-0-415-43469-0 (pbk)
ISBN13: 978-0-203-93575-0 (ebk)

CONTENTS

TABLES AND FIGURES

TABLES

FIGURES

NOTES ON CONTRIBUTORS

Vasilios (Bill) Baltzopoulos is a Professor of Musculoskeletal Biomechanics at the Manchester Metropolitan University. His main research interests focus on joint and muscle-tendon function and loading in both normal and pathological conditions, measurement of muscle strength and biomechanical modelling and processing techniques.

Roger M. Bartlett is Professor of Sports Biomechanics in the School of Physical Education, University of Otago, New Zealand. He is an Invited Fellow of the International Society of Biomechanics in Sports (ISBS) and European College of Sports Sciences, and an Honorary Fellow of the British Association of Sport and Exercise Sciences, of which he was Chairman from 1991–4. Roger is currently editor of the journal *Sports Biomechanics*.

Adrian Burden is a Principal Lecturer in Biomechanics at Manchester Metropolitan University where he is also the Learning & Teaching co-ordinator in the Department of Exercise and Sport Science. His main interests lie in the application of surface electromyography in exercise, clinical and sport settings, and he has run workshops on the use of electromyography for the British Association of Sport and Exercise Sciences.

John H. Challis obtained both his B.Sc. (Honours) and Ph.D. from Loughborough University of Technology. From Loughborough he moved to the University of Birmingham (UK), where he was a lecturer (human biomechanics). In 1996 he moved to the Pennsylvania State University, where he conducts his research in the Biomechanics Laboratory. His research focuses on the coordination and function of the musculo-skeletal system, and data collection and processing methods.

Mark A. King is a Senior Lecturer in Sports Biomechanics at Loughborough University. His research focuses on computer simulation of dynamic jumps, subject-specific parameter determination, racket sports and bowling in cricket.

Mark Lake is currently a Reader in Biomechanics at Liverpool John Moores University. His research interests lie in the area of lower limb biomechanics during sport and exercise with investigations of basic lower extremity function as well as applied aspects relating to sports footwear and injury prevention. He acts as a consultant for several sports shoe manufacturers and is a member of the International Technical Group for Footwear Biomechanics.

Adrian Lees is Professor of Biomechanics and Deputy Director of the Research Institute for Sport and Exercise Sciences. His research interests cover both sport and rehabilitation biomechanics. He has a particular interest in sport technique and its application to soccer and the athletic jump events. He is Chair of the World Commission of Sports Biomechanics Steering Group for Science and Racket Sports. He has also developed and conducted research programmes into wheelchair performance and amputee gait.

Clare E. Milner is an Assistant Professor in the Exercise Science Program of the Department of Exercise, Sport, and Leisure Studies at the University of Tennessee, where she specializes in biomechanics. Her research interests focus on the biomechanics of lower extremity injury and rehabilitation, in particular the occurrence of stress fractures in runners and the quality of walking gait following joint replacement surgery.

David R. Mullineaux is an Assistant Professor at the University of Kentucky, USA. He has made several transitions between academia and industry gaining experience of teaching, consulting and researching in biomechanics and research methods in the UK and USA. His research interest in data analysis techniques has been applied to sport and exercise science, animal science, and human and veterinary medicine.

Carl J. Payton is a Senior Lecturer in Biomechanics at Manchester Metropolitan University. He is High Performance Sport Accredited by the British Association of Sport and Exercise Sciences. His research and scientific support interests are in sports performance, with a particular focus on the biomechanics of elite swimmers with a disability.

Maurice R. (Fred) Yeadon is Professor of Computer Simulation in Sport at Loughborough University. His research interests encompass simulation, motor control, aerial sports, gymnastics and athletics.

CHAPTER 1

INTRODUCTION

Roger M. Bartlett

BACKGROUND AND OVERVIEW

This edition of the 'BASES Biomechanics Guidelines', as they have become almost affectionately known, is an exciting development for the Association, being the first edition to be published commercially. Many changes have taken place in sports biomechanics since the previous edition (Bartlett, 1997) a decade ago. Not only have the procedures used for data collection and analysis in sport and exercise biomechanics continued to expand and develop but also the theoretical grounding of sport and exercise biomechanics has become sounder, if more disparate than formerly.

The collection and summarising of information about our experimental and computational procedures are still, as in earlier editions (Bartlett, 1989; 1992; 1997), very important and we need continually to strive for standardisation of both these procedures and how research studies are reported so as to enable comparisons to be made more profitably between investigations. Most of the chapters that follow focus on these aspects of our activities as sport and exercise biomechanists.

Carl Payton covers all aspects of videography, usually called video analysis in the UK, in Chapter 2. One major change since the previous edition of these guidelines is that cinematography has been almost completely supplanted by videography, despite the considerable drawbacks of the latter particularly in sampling rate and image resolution. Automatic marker-tracking systems have become commonplace in sport and exercise biomechanics research, if not yet in our scientific support work because of the need for body markers and the difficulty of outdoor use. This is reflected in a complete chapter (Chapter 3), contributed by Clare Milner, covering on-line motion analysis systems, whereas they were covered in an 'odds and ends' chapter in the previous edition. I find this new chapter one of the easiest to read in this volume, a tribute to the author as the subject matter is complex.

Image-based motion analysis remains by far and away the most important 'tool' that we use in our work. Important and up-to-date chapters cover other aspects of our experimental work. Adrian Lees and Mark Lake report on force and pressure measuring systems (Chapter 4), Adrian Burden on surface electromyography (Chapter 5), and Vasilios Baltzopoulos on isokinetic dynamometry (Chapter 6). With the loss of the general chapter of the previous edition, other experimental aspects of biomechanics that are peripheral to sport and exercise biomechanics do not feature here. Multiple-image still photography has vanished both from the book and from our practice; accelerometry fails to appear, although it is increasingly used by other biomechanists, mainly because it is a very difficult technique to use successfully in the fast movements that dominate sport; electrogoniometry is not here either as we do not often use it.

In these empirically based chapters, the authors have sought to include an introduction and rationale for the data collection techniques and a discussion of equipment considerations. They have also tried to provide practical, bullet-pointed guidelines on how to collect valid, reliable data and practical advice on how to process, analyse, interpret and present the collected data. Finally, they include bullet-pointed guidelines on what to include in a written report, and follow-up references.

John Challis contributes an important chapter on data processing and error estimation (Chapter 7) and David Mullineaux one on research design and statistics (Chapter 8). One of the most appealing and inventive aspects of this book is the inclusion of a 'theoretical' chapter; Maurice ('Fred') Yeadon and Mark King's chapter (Chapter 9) on computer simulation modelling in sport is an important step forward for this book.

WHAT SPORT AND EXERCISE BIOMECHANISTS DO

The British Association of Sport and Exercise Sciences (BASES) accredits biomechanists in one of two categories: research and scientific support services. Sport and exercise biomechanists also fulfil educational and consultancy roles. These four categories of professional activity are outlined in the following sub-sections and broadly cover how we apply our skills. Not all sport and exercise biomechanists are actively involved in all four of these roles; for example, some of us are accredited by BASES for either research or scientific support services rather than for both.

Research

Both fundamental and applied research are important for the investigation of problems in sport and exercise biomechanics. Applied research provides the necessary theoretical grounds to underpin education and scientific support services; fundamental research allows specific applied research to be developed. Sport and exercise biomechanics requires a research approach based on a mixture of experimentation and theoretical modelling. Many of the problems of the experimental approach are outlined in Chapters 2 to 8.

Scientific support services

It is now undoubtedly true that more sport and exercise biomechanists in the UK provide scientific support services to sports performers and coaches, and clients in the exercise and health sector, than engage in full-time research. In this 'support' role, we biomechanists use our scientific knowledge for the benefit of our clients. This usually involves undertaking a needs analysis to ascertain the client's requirements, followed by the development and implementation of an intervention strategy. First, we seek to understand the problem and all of its relevant aspects. Then the appropriate qualitative or quantitative analytical techniques are used to deliver the relevant scientific support: in scientific support work, these are far more often qualitative than quantitative, although this is not reflected in the contents of this book. Sport and exercise biomechanists then provide careful interpretation of the data from our analyses, translating our science into 'user friendly' terms appropriate to each problem and each client. Increasingly, this scientific support role for sport and exercise biomechanists has a multi-disciplinary or inter-disciplinary focus. This may involve the person concerned having a wider role than simply biomechanics, for example by also undertaking notational analysis of games as a performance analyst or advising on strength and conditioning. It may also involve biomechanists working in inter-disciplinary teams with other sport and exercise scientists, medical practitioners or sports technologists.

Education

As educators, sport and exercise biomechanists are primarily involved in informing the widest possible audience of how biomechanics can enhance understanding of, for example, sports performance, causes of injury, injury prevention, sport and exercise equipment, and the physical effects of the environment. Many people benefit from this education, including coaches and performers at all standards, teachers, medical and paramedical practitioners, exercise and health professionals, leisure organisers and providers, national governing body administrators and the media.

Consultancy

A demand also exists for services, usually on a consultancy basis, from sport and exercise biomechanists, scientists or engineers with detailed specialist knowledge, experience or equipment. This arises, for example, in relation to sport and exercise equipment design or injury diagnostics. The procedure for obtaining such services normally involves consultation with an experienced sport and exercise biomechanist in the first instance.

ANALYSIS SERVICES

Sport and exercise biomechanists offer various types of analysis to suit the needs of each application and its place in the overall framework of biomechanical activities. These can be categorised as qualitative or quantitative analysis as follows.

Qualitative analysis

Qualitative analysis has become more widely used by sport and exercise biomechanists as our role has moved from being researchers to being involved, either partly or as a full-time occupation, in a scientific support role with various clients in sport and exercise, including sports performers and coaches. Some of us have also, along with new theoretical approaches to our discipline such as dynamical systems theory, started to reappraise the formerly narrow concept of what qualitative analysis involves (for a further discussion of these new approaches in the context of an undergraduate textbook, see Bartlett, 2007).

Qualitative analysis is still used in teaching or coaching to provide the learner with detailed feedback to improve performance and, in the context of analysing performance, to differentiate between individuals when judging performance, in gymnastics for example. It is also used in descriptive comparisons of performance, such as in qualitative gait analysis. Qualitative analysis can only be provided successfully by individuals who have an excellent understanding of the specific sport or exercise movements and who can liaise with a particular client group. Such liaison requires a positive, ongoing commitment by the individuals involved. Although qualitative analysis has been seen in the past as essentially descriptive, this has changed with the increasing focus on the evaluation, diagnosis and intervention stages of the scientific support process, and may change further with new interpretations of the movement patterns on which the qualitative analyst should focus (Bartlett, 2007).

Quantitative analysis

The main feature of quantitative analysis is, naturally, the provision of quantitative information, which has been identified as relevant to the sport or exercise activity being studied. The information required may involve variables such as linear and angular displacements, velocities, accelerations, forces, torques, energies and powers; these may be used for detailed technical analysis of a particular movement. Increasingly, sport and exercise biomechanics are looking at continuous time-series data rather than discrete measures. Furthermore, we study movement coordination through, for example, angle-angle diagrams, phase planes and relative phase, often underpinned by dynamical systems theory; hopefully, by the next edition of this book, these approaches will be sufficiently developed and standardised to merit a chapter.

Many data are often available to the sport and exercise biomechanist, so that careful selection of the data to be analysed is required and some data reduction will usually be needed. The selection of important data may be based on previous studies that have, for example, correlated certain variables with an appropriate movement criterion; this selection is greatly helped by previous experience. The next stage may involve biomechanical profiling, in which a movement is characterised in a way that allows comparison with previous performances of that movement by the same person or by other people. This obviously requires a pre-established database and some conceptual model of the movement being investigated.

Good quantitative analysis requires rigorous experimental design and methods (Chapter 8). It also often requires sophisticated equipment, as dealt with in Chapters 2–6. Finally, an analysis of the effects of errors in the data is of great importance (Chapter 7).

PROCEDURAL MATTERS

Ethics

Ethical principles for the conduct of research with humans must be adhered to and laboratory and other procedures must comply with the appropriate code of safe practice. These issues are now addressed by the BASES Code of Conduct (Appendix 1). Most institutions also have Research Ethics Committees that consider all matters relating to research with humans. Ethical issues are particularly important when recording movements of minors and the intellectually disadvantaged; however, ethical issues still arise, even when video recording performances in the public domain, such as at sports competitions.

Pre-analysis preparation

It is essential for the success of any scientific support project that mutual respect exists between the client group and the sport and exercise scientists involved. The specific requirements of the study to be undertaken must be discussed and the appropriate analysis selected. In qualitative studies using only video cameras, it is far more appropriate to conduct filming in the natural environment, such as a sports competition or training, instead of a controlled laboratory or field setting. Decisions must also be made about the experimental design, habituation and so on.

Any special requirements must be communicated to the client group well beforehand. Unfamiliarity with procedures may cause anxiety, particularly at first. This will be most noticeable when performing with some equipment encumbrance, as with electromyography or body markers for automatic-tracking systems, or in an unfamiliar environment such as on a force platform. Problems can even arise when there is no obvious intrusion, as with video, if the person involved is aware of being studied. This problem can only be solved by unhurried habituation to the experimental conditions and by adequate explanation of the proposed procedures and the objectives. A quiet, reassuring atmosphere is a prerequisite for competent assessment in an unfamiliar laboratory environment.

Where analyses are repeated at regular intervals, conditions should be kept constant unless the purpose of the study dictates otherwise, as when comparing movements in competition and training. It may be appropriate to consider increasing the frequency of analysis to improve reliability and repeatability, but not to the detriment of the people involved. The programme must be planned in full collaboration with the client group.

Detailed reporting

The standard of reporting of research in sport and exercise biomechanics is often inadequate. It can be argued that the lack of international agreement on the reporting of research has retarded the development of sport and exercise biomechanics and that a need still remains to standardise such reporting. The overriding principle in reporting our work should be, that all relevant details that are necessary to permit a colleague of equal technical ability to replicate the study, must be included. The details should be provided either explicitly or by clear and unambiguous reference to standard, agreed texts or protocols – such as the chapters of this book. This principle should be followed for all experimental procedures, methods and protocols, the data reduction and computational methods, and the reasons for, and justification of, the statistical techniques used. Although it could be argued that reports of analyses carried out for scientific support purposes do not need to include experimental detail and research design, the principle of replicability should always take precedence and such information should be referenced if not included.

Within our reports, we should evaluate the validity, reliability and objectivity of the methods used and of the results obtained. Single trial studies can no longer be supported, given the increasing evidence of the importance and functionality of movement variability in sports movements (see also Chapter 8). Due consideration should be given to estimation of the uncertainty, or error, in all measured variables; this is particularly important where inter- or intra-person comparisons are made and becomes highly problematic in quantitative studies in which body markers are not used (see, for example, Bartlett *et al.*, 2006). The results of the study should be fully evaluated; all limitations, errors, or assumptions made at any stage of the experimental or analytical process should be frankly reported. The fact that informed consent was obtained from all participants should always be reported for ethical reasons.

Although the reporting of research studies in sport and exercise biomechanics should always follow the above guidelines, studies undertaken for coaches, athletes and other client groups may also need to be governed by the principle of confidentiality (see, for example, MacAuley and Bartlett, 2000). Sport and exercise biomechanists should discuss this in advance with their clients. As scientists we should encourage the publication of important scientific results. However, it will often be necessary to suppress the identity of the participants in the study. There may be occasions when, for example, a coach or athlete requests that the results of the study should not be communicated in any form to other coaches and athletes. In such cases, biomechanists should seek a moratorium on publication of no more than four years, with the freedom to publish after that time. It is wise to have such agreements recorded.

REFERENCES

Bartlett, R.M. (1989) *Biomechanical Assessment of the Elite Athlete*, Leeds: British Association of Sports Sciences.

Bartlett, R.M. (ed.) (1992) *Biomechanical Analysis of Performance in Sport*, Leeds: British Association of Sport and Exercise Sciences.

Bartlett, R.M. (ed.) (1997) *Biomechanical Analysis of Movement in Sport and Exercise*, Leeds: British Association of Sport and Exercise Sciences.

Bartlett, R.M. (2007) *Introduction to Sports Biomechanics: Analysing Human Movement Patterns*, London: Routledge.

Bartlett, R.M., Bussey, M. and Flyger, N. (2006) 'Movement variability cannot be determined reliably from no-marker conditions', *Journal of Biomechanics*, 39: 3076–3079.

MacAuley, D. and Bartlett, R.M. (2000) 'The British Olympic Association's Position Statement of Athlete Confidentiality', *Journal of Sports Sciences*, 18: 69. (Published jointly in the British Journal of Sports Medicine.)

CHAPTER 2

MOTION ANALYSIS USING VIDEO

Carl J. Payton

INTRODUCTION

For many decades, cinematography was the most popular measurement technique for those involved in the analysis of human motion. Cine cameras have traditionally been considered superior to video cameras because of their much greater picture resolution and higher frame rates. However, over the last decade, considerable advances have been made in video technology which now make video an attractive alternative to cine. Modern video cameras are now able to deliver excellent picture quality (although still not quite as good as cine) and high-speed models can achieve frames rates at least comparable to high-speed cine cameras. Unlike cine film, most video recording involves no processing time and the recorded images are available for immediate playback and analysis. Video tapes are very inexpensive when compared to the high cost of purchasing and processing of cine film. The significant improvements made in video camera technology, coupled with a substantial fall in price of the hardware over the past decade, has led to cine cameras becoming virtually redundant in sport and exercise biomechanics.

Video recordings of sport and exercise activities are usually made by biomechanists in order to undertake a detailed analysis of an individual's movement patterns. Although on-line systems (Chapter 3) provide an attractive alternative to video, as a method of capturing motion data, video motion analysis has a number of practical advantages over on-line motion analysis including:

- Low cost – video analysis systems are generally considerably cheaper than on-line systems.
- Minimal interference to the performer – video analysis can be conducted without the need for any disturbance to the performer, e.g. attachment of reflective markers.

- Flexibility – video analysis can be used in environments where some on-line systems would be unable to operate effectively, e.g. outdoors, underwater, in competition.
- Allows visual feedback to the performer – video cameras provide a permanent record of the movement that can be viewed immediately. On-line systems do not generally record the image of the performer.

Given the advantages listed above, video analysis will remain, for the foreseeable future, an important method of analysing technique in sport and exercise. Video analysis of a person's technique may be qualitative or quantitative in nature. Qualitative analysis involves a detailed, systematic and structured observation of the performer's movement pattern. The video image is displayed on a TV monitor or computer screen and observed in real-time, slow motion and frame-by-frame. Often, multiple images, e.g. front and side views, are displayed simultaneously to allow a more complete analysis to be undertaken. The purpose of this type of analysis is often to establish the quality of the movement being observed in order to provide some feedback to the performer. It may also be used as a means of identifying the key performance parameters that need to be quantified and monitored in future analyses.

Quantitative analysis involves taking detailed measurements from the video recording to enable key performance parameters to be quantified. This approach requires more sophisticated hardware and software than for a qualitative analysis and it is vital to follow the correct data capture and data processing procedures. Quantitative analysis can be time-consuming as it often involves manually digitising a number of body landmarks (typically eighteen or more points for a full body model) over a large number of video images. Typical landmarks selected for digitisation are those assumed to represent joint centres of rotation (e.g. knee joint centre), segmental endpoints (e.g. end of foot), or external objects (e.g. a sports implement). Two-dimensional co-ordinates resulting from the digitising process are then scaled and smoothed before being used to calculate linear and angular displacement-time histories. Additional kinematic information (velocities and accelerations) is obtained by computing the first and second time derivatives of these displacement data. However, the accuracy of these derivatives will be severely compromised unless the appropriate data processing techniques are used (discussed in Chapter 7). The kinematic information obtained from video can be used to quantify key performance parameters (e.g. a take-off angle during a jump). Such parameters can then be compared between performers (e.g. novice vs. elite), within performers (e.g. fatigued vs. non-fatigued), or monitored over a period of time (e.g. to evaluate the effects of training over a season).

In order to understand the underlying causes of a given sport or exercise technique, more detailed quantitative analyses are often undertaken. The most common approach is that of inverse dynamics (discussed in Chapter 9). This method involves computing kinetic information on the performer (e.g. net joint reaction forces and net moments) from kinematic information obtained through video, or some other form of motion analysis. The inverse dynamics computational procedures require second time-derivative data, i.e. linear and angular accelerations, for the body segments being analysed, and also require valid body segment inertia data (e.g. mass and moment of inertia). The calculated joint moments and forces can be subject to significant errors unless great care is taken to minimise the error in the kinematic and inertia data.

The interpretation of the results of an inverse dynamics analysis is not as straightforward as for a kinematic analysis. Inverse dynamics provides an insight into the net effect of all the muscles crossing a joint, but it does not allow the computation of bone contact forces or the torque produced by individual muscles, or muscle groups, around the joint. Although there are a number of limitations to the inverse dynamics approach (e.g. Winter, 1990), the method can still provide the biomechanist with a much better understanding of the musculo-skeletal forces and torques acting during a sport or exercise activity, than could be obtained from an analysis of the movement patterns alone.

EQUIPMENT CONSIDERATIONS

Selection of the appropriate equipment is important when undertaking a motion analysis study using video. The key components of a video motion analysis system are:

- Video camera – to capture images of the movement;
- Recording and storage device – to record and store the images from the camera. This may be an integral part of the video camera itself (camcorder) or an external unit, e.g. hard-disc;
- Playback system – to allow the video images to be viewed for qualitative or quantitative analysis;
- Co-ordinate digitiser – to allow measurements to be taken from the video images;
- Processing and analysis software – to enable the user to quantify selected parameters of the movement.

Video cameras

When selecting a video camera with the intention of undertaking a biome-chanical analysis of a sport or exercise activity, the important features to consider are:

- picture quality
- frame rate (sampling frequency)
- manual high-speed shutter
- manual aperture adjustment
- light sensitivity
- gen-lock capability
- recording medium (e.g. tape, hard drive).

Picture quality

A video image is made up of a two dimensional array of dots called pixels. A full video image or frame consists of two halves or fields. One field is made up of the odd-numbered horizontal lines of pixels, the other is made up of the even-numbered lines. Video cameras capture an image using one of two methods: interlaced scan or progressive scan. Cameras that use the interlace technique record one field first, followed by the second, and so on. A progressive scan camera records a complete frame and the two fields that comprise this frame are identical. Some cameras have the facility to capture images in either format. With progressive scan, the option to analyse a movement at 50 Hz, by displaying individual video fields, is lost. The number and size of pixels making up a video image determine the resolution of the picture and this, to a large extent, determines the picture quality.

There are a number of different world standards for video equipment; this can sometimes lead to problems of compatibility. For example, a digital video camera purchased in the USA, may not be compatible with a UK sourced DV player. The phase alternating line (PAL) standard is used in Western Europe (except France), Australia and much of East Africa, India and China. Sequential Couleur Avec Mémoire (SECAM) is the standard found in France and Eastern European countries. Both PAL and SECAM video have 625 horizontal lines of pixels. This is referred to as the vertical resolution. National Television Standards Committee (NTSC) is the standard adopted in North America and Japan, and has 525 lines. The maximum vertical resolution of a video image is therefore essentially limited by the video standard used. It should be noted that the vertical resolution of a displayed image might be considerably lower than these figures, depending on the specification of the video equipment used. Picture quality is also influenced by the horizontal resolution of the video. This refers to the number of pixels per horizontal line.

In the past couple of years a new video format called HDV has emerged on the domestic market and is likely to supercede existing standards. The HDV format allows high definition (HD) video images to be recorded and played back on DV tape. HDV video cameras are now commercially available at very affordable prices and the images produced by these cameras have a vertical resolution of either 720 or 1080 lines. When purchasing an HDV camera, it is important to check what mode(s) it can record and playback in (interlaced: 720i/1080i or progressive: 720p/1080p) to ensure that it is compatible with, for example, the display device. Within each of the world video standards just described, there are a number of video recording formats available and these have varying resolutions:

- VHS, VHS-C and 8mm formats each deliver around 240–260 horizontal lines.
- S-VHS, S-VHS-C and Hi-8 video provide around 400 horizontal lines.
- Digital 8 and miniDV deliver at least 500 horizontal lines.
- High Definition (HD) video gives either 720 or 1080 horizontal lines (with either 1280 or 1920 pixels per line).

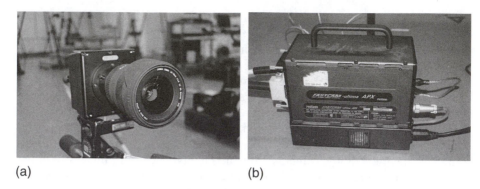

(a)   (b)

Figure 2.1   (a) High-speed video camera (Photron Fastcam Ultima APX) capable of frame rates up to 2000 Hz at full resolution (1024 × 1024 pixels); (b) Camera Processor Unit

Some specialist video cameras (e.g. Photron Fastcam Ultima APX in Figure 2.1) can record images with resolutions higher than those described above. It should be noted that even within a given recording format, e.g. miniDV, the quality of the video image can vary considerably. The resolution of the camera is largely influenced by the quality of its image sensor – the component that converts the light from the object into an electrical signal. The most common type of image sensor is the charge-coupled device (CCD). Most domestic video cameras have a single CCD chip, but some higher quality models have three CCDs (one for each of the primary colours), which result in an improved picture quality. An alternative to the CCD is the complimentary metal oxide semiconductor (CMOS) image sensor. This sensor requires far less power than a CCD and is now used in some standard and high-speed video cameras.

The specification of the camera lens is an important factor in determining picture quality. Digital video cameras will have both an optical zoom range, e.g. 20× and a digital zoom range, e.g. 400×. It is important to note that once a camera is zoomed in beyond the range of its optical system, the picture quality will drastically reduce and will be unsuitable for quantitative analysis. Accessory telephoto lenses can be used to increase the optical zoom of a digital video camera and avoid this problem. They also allows the user to increase the camera-to-subject distance, whilst maintaining the desired image size. This will reduce the perspective error although it should be noted that the addition of a telephoto lens will reduce the amount of light reaching the camera's image sensor. It is important to check how well a telephoto lens performs at the limits of the optical zoom, as this is where image distortion will be most pronounced. Wide-angle lenses can be fitted to video cameras to increase the field of view for a given camera–subject distance. However, such lenses tend to produce considerable image distortion and have limited applications in quantitative analyses.

Frame rate (sampling frequency)

In video capture, the term 'frame' refers to a complete image captured at an instant in time (Greaves, 1995). Thus the frame rate of a video camera refers to the number of full images it captures per second (this is often referred to as the sampling frequency of the camera). Standard PAL video cameras have a frame rate of 25 Hz, whereas NTSC cameras have a frame rate of 30 Hz. If the camera captures using the interlaced scan method, each video frame will be comprised of two video fields (an A and B field). For a video image with a vertical resolution of 480 lines, each field would consist of 240 lines, one field comprised of the odd lines, the other of the even lines. With the appropriate hardware or software, it is possible to display the video fields separately and sequentially thus enabling measurements to be taken at 1/50 of a second increments (or 1/60 of a second for NTSC), but at reduced resolution.

For some sport and exercise activities, the frame rate of conventional video cameras will be too low and a high-speed video camera may be required. High-speed video cameras, as with conventional video cameras, can be analogue or digital (see Greaves, 1995 for more detail). Although video cameras with frame rates beyond 2000 Hz are commercially available, cameras with rates of 100–500 Hz are generally adequate for most sport and exercise biomechanics applications. Although some early high-speed video cameras recorded to tape (e.g. Peak Performance HSC 200 PS), most models now either record the images to RAM (e.g. Photron Fastcam Ultima APX shown in Figure 2.1) or direct to a computer hard drive via a Firewire (IEEE) port (e.g. Basler 602f 100 Hz camera).

One of the major limitations of high-speed cameras that record to RAM is the limited recording time available. For example, a high-speed video camera with a storage capacity of 8 Gb, recording with a resolution of 1024 × 1024 at 2000 Hz, provides a maximum recording duration of approximately three seconds.

High speed shutter

For most biomechanical applications, a video camera equipped with a high-speed shutter is essential. The shutter is the component of a camera that controls the amount of time the camera's image sensor (e.g. CCD, CMOS) is exposed to light. Modern video cameras use electronic shuttering, which involves activating or deactivating the image sensor for a specified time period, as each video field is sampled. When recording movement using a low shutter speed, the image sensor is exposed to the light passing through the camera lens for a relatively long period of time; this can result in a blurred or streaked image being recorded. The extent of the blurring would depend on the speed of the movement being analysed.

It is important that a video camera has a manual shutter speed option. This allows the user to select a 'shutter speed' (this term is a misnomer as it represents the time the shutter is open) that is appropriate for the activity that is being analysed, and the prevalent lighting conditions (see Data Collection Procedures section of this chapter). Typically, a video camera will offer shutter speeds ranging from 1/60–1/4000 of a second. It should be noted that not all video cameras offer a manual shutter function. Camera models that incorporate a Sports Mode function should be avoided because the shutter speed associated with this is often inadequate for fast-moving activities.

Manual iris and low-light sensitivity

The iris is the element of the camera's lens system that controls the aperture (the adjustable gap in the iris) in order to regulate the amount of light falling on the image sensor. If too much light is permitted to pass through the lens (large aperture), for too long, the result will be an overexposed image. If too little light passes through the lens (small aperture), the image will be underexposed. Video cameras generally have automatic aperture control that continually adjusts to ensure the image is correctly exposed. Some camera models have a manual override that allows the user to specify the aperture setting. This is sometimes necessary when conducting biomechanical analyses. For example, when a high shutter speed setting is needed in low light conditions, the iris aperture would have to be opened wider than it would be in automatic mode. The drawback of doing this is the increased noise level in the image, which results in a more 'grainy' picture.

Video cameras each have a minimum light level that they require in order to produce an image. This level is expressed in *lux*. A camera with a minimum illumination value of 1 lux will perform better in low light conditions than one with a 3 lux rating.

Gen-lock capability

For three-dimensional video analysis, it is desirable for the activation of the shutters of the two (or more) cameras to be perfectly synchronised, that is, for the cameras to be gen-locked. This involves physically linking the cameras with a gen-lock cable. Unfortunately, most standard video camcorders do not have the facility to be gen-locked, although some more expensive models do offer this feature (e.g. Canon XL H1 HDV 1080i camera). If video cameras cannot be gen-locked, the two-dimensional co-ordinates obtained from each of the camera views must be synchronised by interpolating the data and then shifting one data set by the time lag between the camera shutters. The time lag will be no more than half the reciprocal of frame rate of the camera (e.g. at 25 Hz, the time lag will be <20 ms). The simplest method of determining the time lag is to have a timing device in the field of view of all cameras. Where this is not possible, for example when filming at a competition, a method involving a mathematical analysis of the co-ordinates of all the digitised body landmarks, has been proposed (Yeadon and King, 1999). Alternatively, certain commercial video capture and analysis software packages, for example SIMI°Motion, will automatically measure the time lag between camera shutters, if the video images from the cameras are simultaneously captured to a hard drive, via the software, in real-time. The software will also interpolate and phase shift the two-dimensional co-ordinates to enable three-dimensional reconstruction to be undertaken.

Recording medium

Images from video cameras have traditionally been recorded onto some form of tape, for example, S-VHS and miniDV. In recent years a number of alternative recording formats have emerged. Video cameras that record straight to a small DVD are more geared toward the home movie-maker, than those wanting to undertake a quantitative analysis of movement. More viable alternatives to tape recording cameras are those with built-in memory. This may be in the form of a hard disc drive (HDD), internal memory (D-RAM) or Flash Memory.

Recording and storage device

A video camera that records the images to tape provides the user with a number of options, depending on what type of analysis they are performing. For a qualitative analysis, the recorded movement can be viewed directly from the videotape in real-time, slow motion or as a still image, using an appropriate video playback system, without the need for any computer hardware or software. Alternatively, the user may choose to capture the video images from the tape to a computer hard drive, where they are stored in the form of a video file (e.g. AVI, MPEG, etc.). This is an attractive option as, with the aid of appropriate software, images can be presented in ways that are not easily achievable when playing back directly from tape, for example, the display of multiple video clips simultaneously. It also enables a quantitative analysis to be undertaken, if appropriate digitising, processing and analysis software is installed.

Video images that are recorded to a camera's hard disc drive (HDD), RAM or Flash Memory are usually transferred subsequently to a computer hard drive, where they can be displayed or processed for quantitative analysis. The process of capturing video images to a computer can either be done in real-time or at some point following the filming session. Which of these approaches is taken will be determined by a number of factors including the specification of the camera and the filming environment. For video cameras that record to tape, or which have their own hard drive or memory, capture to computer can be done post-recording. With the majority of high-speed cameras this is the only option, as the required data transfer rate exceeds the capability of the system. In most situations with standard 50 Hz cameras (and some higher speed cameras), capture of video to computer can be done in real-time. With appropriate software, and the requisite connectivity, video sequences from two or more cameras can be captured simultaneously in real-time. When capturing video images to a computer, the following practical issues need to be considered:

Specification of computer

For real-time video capture from standard digital video cameras, a Firewire IEEE-1394 connection is required (often referred to as DVin or i-Link). If this is not an integral part of the computer, a Firewire hub can be connected via the USB or PCI port. Alternatively, a PCMCIA Firewire card can be used (for laptops). For some high-speed digital camera models, a USB 2.0 or Ethernet port is required to download video data. For capture from an analogue source, some form of video capture board is needed. This must be able to capture in a file format and resolution that is compatible with the digitising software.

All modern computers will have a sufficiently fast processor and adequate RAM to manage the data transfer rates involved in standard digital video capture (Firewire supports transfer rates up to 400 Mbit/s which is more than adequate for DV video). An important consideration is the available hard disc space. The size of an uncompressed five second video file captured at a resolution of 720×526 pixels is about 18 Mb. Four minutes of uncompressed digital video will therefore require almost 1 Gb of hard disc space.

Capture software

Capture software is used to convert or encode the video to the required file format or 'codec'. The capture settings used within the software are critical. For quantitative analysis, the format of the captured video file (e.g. AVI, MPEG) must be compatible with the digitising software. The user should generally capture in the highest quality available. Image quality should not be compromised for the sake of file size, by using high-compression formats, unless absolutely necessary.

Video playback system

A video playback system is required to display the video images for qualitative or quantitative analysis. The system should be capable of displaying 'flicker free' still images. It should also allow video sequences to be played in slow motion and in real-time.

For qualitative analysis, an analogue or digital video player-recorder (VCR) linked to a TV monitor is a viable option. This should be equipped with a jog-shuttle dial to control pause and picture advance functions. For analogue video, such as S-VHS, a four-head VCR is necessary for a stable still image. Some professional grade VCRs will enable individual video fields to be displayed, thus providing the user with 50 images per second (compared with 25 per second on most domestic video players). This facility is important when analysing all but very slow movements. The picture quality on a video monitor is influenced by the quality of the source tape, the specification of video playback device, the type of video cable used to link the playback device to the monitor (in ascending order of quality: composite, S-video, Scart (RGB), component, DVI, HDMI), and the monitor itself.

Traditional CRT monitors generally offer excellent picture resolution but cannot directly display a digital source. LCD Monitors vary in their resolution (e.g. VGA monitor: 640×480; XGA monitor: 1024×768; HD monitor: 1366×768). Some models of LCD monitors can only display analogue sources, some only digital sources, and some can display both.

For quantitative analysis, video playback will be via a laptop or desktop computer. Here, the video data are processed through the computer's graphics card and displayed on the monitor. The quality of the image will be influenced by the specification of the graphics card, the video playback codec, compression settings, monitor resolution, and the digitising software.

Co-ordinate digitiser

To undertake a detailed quantitative analysis, a co-ordinate digitiser is required. This device enables two-dimensional (x, y) co-ordinates of specified points on the video image, for example, anatomical landmarks, to be recorded. Video-based co-ordinate digitisers are essentially software applications that display the still video image on a computer screen and overlay this with a cursor that is manually controlled by the user. The most important consideration when selecting a video digitising system is its measurement resolution. This refers to the minimum separation between two points on the screen that the system is able to detect. The digitiser resolution affects the level of precision to which the co-ordinates can be measured. Current video-based digitising systems offer considerably higher measurement resolutions than were available in early systems. This is achieved through a combination of zoom and a sub-pixel cursor. For example, QUINTIC Biomechanics 9.03 (Quintic Consultancy Ltd, Coventry, UK) displays the non-magnified standard video image at a resolution of 720 (horizontal) by 526 (vertical). This resolution can be increased linearly using the software's zoom function (up to a maximum of $10\times$). At a $3\times$ magnification, this provides a measurement resolution of approximately 0.05%. The TARGET video digitising system developed at Loughborough University combines a $4\times$ magnification with a sub-pixel cursor to produce a digitising resolution of $12,288 \times 9,216$ (Kerwin, 1995). It should be noted that, unless the resolution of the captured video is high, the image will become very 'pixilated' at high magnifications.

DATA COLLECTION PROCEDURES

When conducting a quantitative video analysis, certain procedures must be followed carefully, at both the video recording and digitising stages, to minimise the systematic and random errors in the digitised co-ordinates. Even when undertaking a qualitative video analysis, many of the video recording procedures are still pertinent as they will help to obtain a high quality video record of the performance.

Quantitative video analysis may be two-dimensional or three-dimensional. The former approach is much simpler, but it assumes that the movement being analysed is confined to a single, pre-defined plane – the plane of motion. Any measurements taken of movements outside this plane will be subject to perspective error, thus reducing their accuracy. Even activities that appear to be two-dimensional, such as a walking gait, are likely to involve movements in more than one plane; a two-dimensional analysis would not enable these to be quantified accurately. Three-dimensional analysis enables the true spatial movements of the performer to be quantified. This approach eliminates perspective error, but the video filming and analysis procedures are more complicated, and the equipment requirements are also greater.

Two-dimensional video recording

The following guidelines are designed to minimise the systematic and random errors present in two-dimensional co-ordinates, resulting from the video recording stage. This will increase the accuracy of any parameters subsequently obtained from these co-ordinates. The guidelines are based on those previously reported in Bartlett, 1997b, and in earlier texts (Miller and Nelson, 1973; Smith, 1975).

Equipment set-up

Mount the camera on a stable tripod and avoid panning
The standard approach in a two-dimensional analysis is for the camera to remain stationary as the performer moves through the field of view. This enables the movement of the performer to be determined easily relative to an external frame of reference.

Two-dimensional filming techniques involving panning or tracking cameras have been used when the performance occurs over a long path (for example Gervais *et al.*, 1989; Chow, 1993). As these methods involve the camera moving (rotating or translating) relative to the external frame of reference, mathematical corrections have to be made for this movement if accurate two-dimensional co-ordinates are to be obtained.

Maximise the camera-to-subject distance
The camera must be positioned as far as is practically possible from the performer. This will reduce the perspective error that results from movement outside the plane of performance (see Figure 2.2).

A telephoto zoom lens will enable the camera-to-subject distance to be increased whilst maintaining the desired image size. Note that image quality will be reduced if a digital video camera is positioned beyond the limit of its optical zoom system.

Maximise the image size
To increase the accuracy during digitising, the image of the performer must be as large as possible. Image size is inversely proportional to the field of view of the camera. The camera should therefore only be zoomed out sufficiently for the field of view to encompass the performance path, plus a small margin for error.

For events that occur over long performance paths, e.g. triple jump, a single stationary camera would not provide an image size suitable for

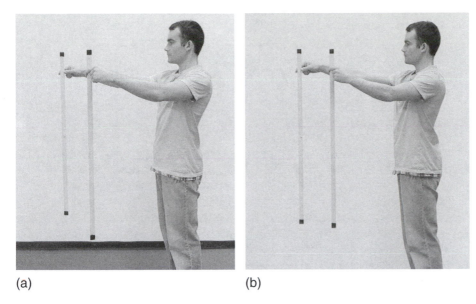

(a)   (b)

Figure 2.2 Apparent discrepancy in the lengths of two identical rods when recorded using a camera-to-subject distance of 3 m (image a) and 20 m (image b). Note that the rods are being held shoulder width apart

quantitative analysis. In such situations, the use of multiple synchronised cameras, or a panning/tracking camera method, would be required.

Focus the camera manually

Most video cameras have an automatic focus system that can be manually overridden. In most situations, the camera should be set in manual focus mode. For a well-focused image, zoom in fully on an object in the plane of motion, manually focus, and zoom out to the required field of view.

Align the optical axis of the camera perpendicular to the plane of motion

Any movements that are performed within a pre-defined plane of motion will not be subject to perspective error at the digitising stage, provided this plane is parallel to the camera image sensor (perpendicular to the camera optical axis). As no human movement is truly planar, it is essential to establish which aspect of the activity is of primary interest and in which plane this occurs. The camera can then be positioned accordingly. Marking a straight line from the camera lens to the geometric centre of the field of view can represent the direction of the optical axis. Various methods can be used to align the optical axis orthogonal to the plane of motion. A common approach is to use right angle triangles (triangles whose sides are in the ratio 3:4:5). Failure to ensure that the optical axis is orthogonal to the plane of motion, even by a few degrees, can have a detrimental effect on the accuracy of the analysis (Brewin and Kerwin, 2003). Even with a correctly aligned camera, movement will inevitably occur outside the plane of motion. The effect on measured angles is illustrated in Figure 2.3.

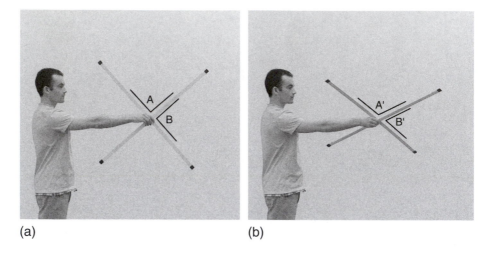

(a)   (b)

Figure 2.3 Distortion of angles when movement occurs outside the plane of motion. The true value of angles A and B is 90° (image a). In image b, angle A appears to be greater than 90° (A′) and angle B appears to be less than 90° (B′), as the frame is no longer in the plane of motion

Record a vertical reference

To enable a true vertical (and horizontal) frame of reference to be established at the digitising stage, a clear vertical reference, such as a plumb line, must be recorded after the camera set-up has been completed. Any good video digitising system will correct for a non-vertically aligned camera, using the co-ordinates of the vertical reference.

Record a scaling object

An object whose dimensions are accurately known must be recorded in the plane of motion. This is to enable image co-ordinates to be transformed to object-space (real world) co-ordinates following the digitising stage. Recording of the scaling object(s) must be done only after the camera set-up is complete.

The use of both horizontal and vertical scaling objects is essential, because the computer may display the image with an aspect ratio (ratio of the width to the height) that distorts it in one dimension. To minimise the error in the scaling process, the dimensions of the scaling objects should be such that they occupy a good proportion of the width and height of the field of view. For a given digitising error, the scaling error will be inversely proportional to the length of the scaling object. For field widths greater than 2–3 m, scaling is usually done using the known distance between two or more reference markers or control points, positioned in the plane of motion.

In some circumstances it is not possible to align the camera optical axis correctly with the plane of motion, for example when filming in a competition. Here, digitisation of a grid of control points, placed in the plane of motion, can be used to correct for the camera misalignment. This method is called *2D-DLT* and has been shown to provide significantly more accurate reconstruction of two-dimensional co-ordinate data than the more commonly used scaling techniques, particularly when the optical axis of the camera is tilted more than a few degrees relative to the plane of motion (Brewin and Kerwin, 2003).

Select an appropriate shutter speed and aperture

In activities such as running, jumping, throwing and kicking, it is the most distal body segments, the hands and feet, which move the quickest. A shutter speed should be selected that is sufficient to provide a non-blurred image of the fastest moving body segments (or sports implements). The choice of shutter speed depends on the type of activity being recorded. For slow movements, such as a grande plié in ballet or walking, shutter speeds of 1/150–1/250 of a second should be adequate; for moderately fast activities, such as running or a swimming start, shutter speeds of 1/350–1/750 of a second are more appropriate; for fast activities such as a golf swing or a tennis serve, a shutter speed of 1/1000 of a second or above may be needed.

An increase in shutter speed will always be accompanied by a decrease in image quality, for given lighting conditions and camera aperture setting. To obtain the best possible images at the required shutter speed, sufficient lighting must be provided such that the camera iris aperture does not have to be opened excessively.

Ensure correct lighting of the performer

If filming indoors, floodlights are often needed to achieve the required lighting level. Bartlett, 1997a, suggests that one floodlight positioned perpendicular to the plane of performance, and one to each side at around 30° to the plane, should provide adequate illumination. Filming outdoors in natural daylight is often preferable to filming under artificial lights, but natural light levels are inevitably less predictable. When filming in direct sunlight, the position of the sun will restrict where the camera can be located. The background must provide a good contrast with the performer and be as plain and uncluttered as possible. When filming indoors with floodlighting, a dark, non-reflective background is preferred. Video cameras often have a manually adjustable setting for different light sources (e.g. daylight, fluorescent lamps, sodium or mercury lamps) and white balance, which can be used to enhance the colour rendition.

Select an appropriate frame rate

Standard PAL video cameras have a fixed frame rate of 25 Hz, although this can effectively be doubled, provided the camera uses the interlaced scan method. Most high-speed cameras have adjustable frame rates. The frame rate used will depend on the frequency content of the movement being analysed, and the dependent variables being studied. Sampling Theorum (see Chapter 7 for more detail) states that the sampling frequency (frame rate) must be at least double that of the highest frequency present in the activity itself. In reality, the frame rate should be much higher than this (Challis et al., 1997) suggest 8–10 times higher).

A sufficiently high frame rate will ensure that the instances of maximum and minimum displacement (linear and angular) of a joint or limb, and of other key events in a performance (e.g. heel-strike in running, ball impact in a golf swing) are recorded. An increase in the frame rate will also serve to improve the precision, and therefore the accuracy, of temporal measurements, for example, the phase durations of a movement. This is particularly important where the phases are of short duration, for example, the hitting phase of a tennis serve. Some suggested frame rates for a variety of activities are given below:

- 25–50 Hz – walking, swimming, stair climbing.
- 50–100 Hz – running, shot put, high jump.
- 100–200 Hz – sprinting, javelin throwing, football kick.
- 200–500 Hz – tennis serve, golf swing, parry in fencing.

It should be noted that these frame rates are only offered as a guide. For a given activity, the appropriate frame rate should be determined by the frequency content of the activity and the dependent variables being measured. For example, a quantitative analysis of the interaction between the player's foot and the ball during a football kick would require a frame rate above 1000 Hz, whereas a rate of 25 Hz would be more than adequate for determining the length of the final stride during the approach to the ball. The effect of using different frame rates on the recording of a football kick is shown in Figure 2.4.

Participant preparation and recording trials

The health and safety of the participant is paramount during any testing. Informed consent should always be obtained from the participant (see BASES Code of Conduct in Appendix 1) and completion of a health questionnaire is often required. Sufficient time must be allocated for a warm-up and for the participant to become fully familiar with the testing environment and testing conditions.

The clothing worn by the participant should allow the limbs and body landmarks relevant to the analysis to be seen clearly. The careful placement of small markers on the skin can help the analyst to locate body landmarks during digitising, but the positioning of these markers must be considered carefully. Movement of soft tissue means that surface markers can only ever provide a guide to the structures of the underlying skeleton. Markers are often used to help identify the location of a joint's instantaneous centre of rotation. Whilst a single marker can adequately represent the axis of a simple hinge joint, more complex joints may require more complex marker systems (see Chapter 3 for more detail on marker systems).

The number of trials recorded will depend on the purpose of the analysis and the skill level of the participants. As the movement patterns of skilled performers are likely to be significantly more consistent than those of novice performers (Williams and Ericsson, 2005), they may be required to perform fewer trials in order to demonstrate a typical performance. During the filming it is often useful to record a board in the field of view, showing information such as the date, performer, trial number and condition, and camera settings.

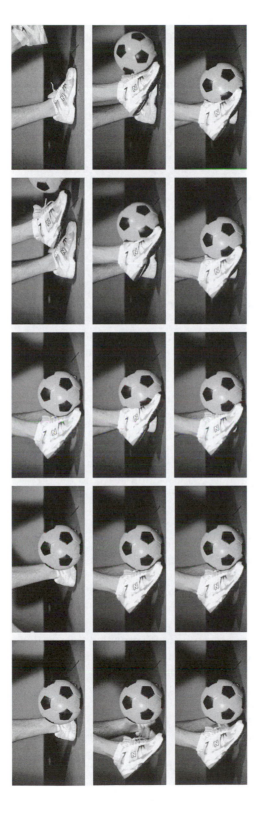

Figure 2.4 The effect of camera frame rate on the recording of a football kick. At 50 Hz (top row) the foot is only seen in contact with the ball for one image; at 250 Hz (middle row) the foot remains in contact for four images; at 1000 Hz (bottom row) the foot is in contact for sixteen images (not all images shown)

Three-dimensional video recording

Many of the procedures described in the previous section for two-dimensional video analysis will also apply when using a three-dimensional approach (selecting an appropriate frame rate, shutter speed and aperture; ensuring correct lighting of the performer; maximising the image size and focusing the camera manually). This section will discuss the main issues that must be considered at the recording stage of a three-dimensional analysis.

Equipment set-up

The essential requirement is to have two or more cameras simultaneously recording the performance, each from a different perspective. The choice of algorithm used to reconstruct the three-dimensional, real world co-ordinates from the two-dimensional image co-ordinates is important as some algorithms place severe restrictions on camera locations.

Some three-dimensional reconstruction algorithms rely on very precise positioning of the cameras relative to one another. For example, the method proposed by Martin and Pongrantz, 1974, requires the optical axes of the cameras to be orthogonally aligned and intersecting. Such methods can involve considerable set-up time and may be impractical to use in some environments, e.g. in sports competitions, as they are too restrictive.

The most widely used three-dimensional reconstruction algorithm used in sport and exercise biomechanics is the Direct Linear Transformation (DLT) algorithm. This approach does not require careful camera alignment and thus allows more flexibility in the choice of camera locations. The DLT method determines a linear relationship between the two-dimensional image co-ordinates of, for example, a body landmark, and the three-dimensional, real world co-ordinates of that landmark. A detailed theoretical background to the DLT algorithm can be found elsewhere (e.g. Abdel-Aziz and Karara, 1971; Miller, Shapiro and McLaughlin, 1980).

To establish the relationship between the two-dimensional image co-ordinates and the three-dimensional real world co-ordinates, an object space or performance volume must be defined using a set of control points whose real world, three-dimensional co-ordinates are known. This is usually achieved using a rigid calibration frame of known dimensions incorporating a set of visible markers such as small spheres (see Figures 2.5 and 2.6). Alternatively, a series of discrete calibration poles can be used, provided their real world co-ordinates have been accurately established using, for example, surveying techniques.

A minimum of six non-coplanar control points is required for the reconstruction of three-dimensional co-ordinates, but 15–20 control points or more is recommended. The control point co-ordinates must be known relative to three orthogonal, intersecting axes, which define a global co-ordinate system or inertial reference system. This reference system is fixed in space and all three-dimensional co-ordinates are derived relative to this. Images of the control points are recorded by each of the cameras being used in the set-up. These are then digitised to produce a set of two-dimensional co-ordinates for

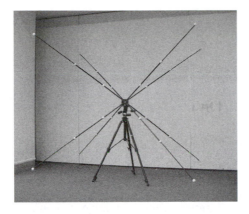

Figure 2.5 Calibration frame (1.60 m × 1.91 m × 2.23 m) with 24 control points (Peak Performance Technologies Inc.)

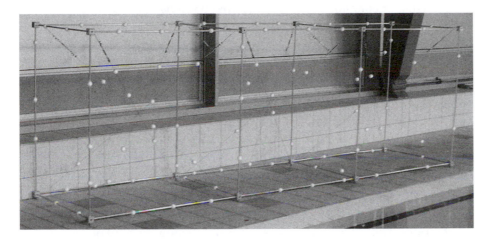

Figure 2.6 Calibration frame (1.0 m × 1.5 m × 4.5 m) with 92 control points (courtesy of Ross Sanders)

each control point from each camera view. These co-ordinates are used to compute the 11 DLT parameters (C_1–C_{11}), which relate to the orientation and position of each of the cameras. For control point #1 with real world, object space co-ordinates (X_1, Y_1, Z_1) and with digitised co-ordinates (x_1, y_1) from camera 1, the DLT equations for that camera are given by equations 2.1 and 2.2.

$$x_1 + C_1X_1 + C_2Y_1 + C_3Z_1 + C_4 + C_9x_1X_1 + C_{10}x_1Y_1 + C_{11}x_1Z_1 = 0 \tag{2.1}$$

$$y_1 + C_5X_1 + C_6Y_1 + C_7Z_1 + C_8 + C_9y_1X_1 + C_{10}y_1Y_1 + C_{11}y_1Z_1 = 0 \tag{2.2}$$

For the minimum of six control points, twelve equations are produced for each camera view. As there are more equations than unknowns, the DLT parameters are obtained by solving the equations using a least-squares technique (Miller, Shapiro and McLaughlin, 1980). With the DLT parameters obtained, the same equations can then be used to obtain the three-dimensional co-ordinates of any marker in the object space, provided the two-dimensional co-ordinates of the marker are known from at least two of the cameras.

When setting up the equipment for three-dimensional analysis the biomechanist should follow the steps in the sub-sections below.

Mount the cameras on stable tripods and avoid panning

The standard approach in a three-dimensional analysis is for the cameras to remain stationary as the performer moves through their field of view. Three-dimensional filming techniques involving panning cameras (e.g. Yu *et al.*, 1993; Yanai *et al.*, 1996) and panning and tilting cameras (e.g. Yeadon, 1989) have been used when the performance occurs over a long path. As these methods involve the cameras moving relative to the global co-ordinate system, a number of fixed reference markers have to be digitised in each video image to correct for the changing orientation of the cameras. An alternative method of establishing the orientation of panning and tilting video cameras was developed by Peak Performance Technologies Inc. This involves the use of instrumented tripod heads, each equipped with two optical encoders, to sense the angular positions of the cameras.

Position the cameras for optimum viewing of body landmarks

Great care should be taken to ensure that the body landmarks of interest (e.g. segment endpoints) remain in view of at least two cameras for the duration of the activity. Inappropriately positioned cameras can result in the analyst having to guess limb positions at certain stages of the movement, which will inevitably compromise the accuracy of the co-ordinate data. Many video motion analysis programmes offer an interpolation function that can predict the co-ordinates of a body landmark that has become obscured. This option should only be used in situations where the landmark is concealed for no more than four or five images and is not reaching a turning point (maximum or minimum) during that period.

Ensure control points are visible to and recorded by all cameras

The control points used to compute the DLT parameters must be clearly visible to each camera. When using a calibration frame, such as the one shown in Figure 2.5, care should be taken to avoid the poles at the rear of the frame being obscured by those in the foreground (or by the tripod). A good contrast between the control points and the background is also essential. It is advisable to record the control points at the start and end of the data collection session. This will allow the analyst to recalibrate if one of the cameras is accidentally moved slightly during the session.

Align the performance with the axes of the global co-ordinate system

The International Society of Biomechanics (ISB) recommends that, where there is an obvious direction of progression, for example in gait, the X-axis of the global co-ordinate system be nominally aligned with this direction.

They propose the use of a right-handed co-ordinate system, with the Y-axis being directed vertically and the Z-axis laterally.

Make provision for shutter synchronisation and event synchronisation

Ideally, the two or more cameras should be gen-locked to ensure their shutters are synchronised. Where this is not possible, the time lag between each of the camera shutters must be determined so the two-dimensional co-ordinates obtained from each camera view can be synchronised (see Video Cameras section in this chapter).

During filming, it is useful to activate an event marker e.g. an LED or strobe light that is visible to all cameras. Such a device can be used to confirm that the first video image digitised from a given camera view corresponds temporally to the first image digitised from all other camera views. Failure to fulfil this requirement will result in erroneous three-dimensional co-ordinates.

Video digitising

The process of obtaining two-dimensional co-ordinates of specified landmarks on the performer, from a video record, may be achieved automatically or manually. Most video motion analysis systems (e.g. APAS, Qualisys, SIMI°Motion) now include software that can automatically track passive markers affixed to the performer. While this facility is clearly an attractive option for the user, it is not always possible or practical to place markers on the performer, e.g. during a sports competition. Even where this is possible, automatic tracking of passive markers can still be problematic, particularly in environments where the contrast level of the marker is variable, e.g. when filming outdoors or underwater.

Manual digitising of a video record requires the biomechanist to visually identify and mark the anatomical sites of interest, frame-by-frame. This process will inevitably introduce some systematic and random errors to the co-ordinate data (see Chapter 7 for more detail). With attention to detail, these errors can be kept to an acceptable level. The following points should be considered when manually digitising a video sequence:

- The same operator should digitise all trials in the study to ensure consistency (reliability) between trials.
- Only ever use skin-mounted markers as a guide. Consider carefully the anatomical landmark being sought. A sound knowledge of the underlying musculo-skeletal system is essential here.
- Great care should be taken when digitising the scaling object or control points. Any measurement error here will introduce a systematic error in the co-ordinate data, and in all variables derived from these.
- On completion of a 3D calibration, check that the 3D reconstruction errors fall within acceptable limits. These errors will depend mainly on the volume of the object-space being calibrated, the quality of the video image and the resolution of the digitiser. As a guide, Sanders et al., 2006,

reported mean RMS reconstruction errors of 3.9 mm, 3.8 mm and 4.8 mm for the *x*, *y* and *z* co-ordinates, respectively, of 30 points distributed throughout the large calibration frame shown in Figure 2.6.

- A representative sequence should be digitised several times by the investigator to establish the intra-operator reliability. Inter-operator reliability (objectivity) should also be determined by having one or more other experienced individuals digitise the same sequence (see Chapter 7 and Atkinson and Nevill, 1998, for more information on assessing measurement reliability).

PROCESSING, ANALYSING AND PRESENTING VIDEO-DERIVED DATA

The video digitising process creates two-dimensional image co-ordinates that are contaminated with high frequency errors (noise). Essentially, what is required next is to: 1) smooth and transform the co-ordinates, so that they are in a form suitable for computing kinematic variables, 2) calculate and display the kinematic variables in a format that allows the user to extract the information required to complete the analysis.

Smoothing and transforming co-ordinates

There are various smoothing methods that can be used to remove the high frequency noise introduced by the digitising process; these fall into three general categories: digital filters, spline fitting and fourier series truncation (Bartlett, 1997a). Failure to smooth co-ordinates sufficiently will lead to high levels of noise in any derived kinematic variables, particularly acceleration. Oversmoothing of the co-ordinates will result in some of the original signal being lost. Selecting the correct smoothing factor, for a given set of co-ordinates, is therefore critically important. Chapter 7 provides a detailed discussion of smoothing methods and presents some practical guidelines for their use. The transformation of image co-ordinates to real world co-ordinates is necessary before any analysis can be undertaken. Procedures for achieving this were discussed earlier in this chapter.

Calculating kinematic variables

The sport and exercise biomechanist is often interested both in the movement patterns of individual body segments, for example in throwing and kicking, and in the overall motion of the performer's centre of mass, for example in a sprint start. Computation of the mass centre location requires a linked-segment model to be defined, and the mass, and mass centre locations, of individual body segments to be determined. Three general methods are used to obtain body segment parameters: regression equations based on measurements taken from cadavers, geometric modelling of the body segments, and the use of imaging devices (Bartlett, 1997a). More detail on these methods can be found in Robertson, 2004. The biomechanist should seek to use segmental inertia data that closely match the physical characteristics of the participants being analysed.

The linear displacement of a body landmark (or mass centre) in one dimension (e.g. x direction) is defined as the change in the relevant scaled co-ordinate of that landmark (Δx) during a specified time period. Resultant linear displacements in two or three dimensions are easily calculated using Pythagoras' theorem. Two-dimensional (planar) angles are obtained from two-dimensional co-ordinates using simple trigonometry. These angles may be relative (e.g. joint angles formed by two adjacent segments) or absolute (e.g. the angle of a segment relative to the vertical). Planar angles are relatively simple to interpret, once the angular conventions adopted by the analysis system have been established. The calculation of relative (joint) angles from three-dimensional co-ordinates is more complex, as is their interpretation. The most common methods used for calculating three-dimensional joint angles in biomechanics are the Euler and Joint Co-ordinate System (JCS) methods. A detailed discussion of these methods is provided by Andrews, 1995.

Linear and angular velocities and accelerations are defined as the first and second time derivatives of the displacement (linear or angular), respectively. These derivatives can be computed either numerically (e.g. finite difference method) or analytically (if the data have been smoothed with mathematical functions). As with displacement, the orthogonal components of velocity and acceleration can analysed separately, or their resultants can be found.

Analysing and presenting video-derived data

In any biomechanical analysis, the selection of dependent variables will be determined by the aim of the study. It is important that the biomechanical variables of interest are identified before undertaking the data collection, as this will influence the methodology used (e.g. 2D vs. 3D; normal vs. high-speed video). When analysing a sport or exercise activity, the use of deterministic models (Hay and Reid, 1982) can help to identify the important movement parameters, as of course can reference to the appropriate research literature.

There are a number of ways of presenting the kinematic data from a video analysis and it is for the individual to decide on the most appropriate presentation format. This will be dictated mainly by the intended destination of the information (e.g. research journal, athlete feedback report). The most common methods of presenting kinematic data are as discrete measures (e.g. peak joint angles) and as time series plots (e.g. hip velocity vs. time). Where the focus of the analysis is on movement co-ordination, the use of angle–angle plots and angle–angular velocity (phase) plots is becoming increasingly popular in sport and exercise biomechanics.

REPORTING A VIDEO MOTION ANALYSIS STUDY

The biomechanist should consider including some or all of the following information when reporting a video-based study.

Participants

- Participant details (age, height, body mass, trained status etc.);
- Method of obtaining informed consent (verbal or written);
- Nature of the warm-up and familiarisation;
- Type of clothing worn, type and position of skin/other markers and the method of locating body landmarks.

Video recording

- Camera and lens type (manufacturer and model) and the recording medium, format and resolution (e.g. HD 720i on to miniDV tape);
- Camera settings (frame rate, shutter speed, iris (f-stop) setting);
- Position of camera(s) relative to the movement being recorded and the field width obtained from each camera (a diagram is useful here);
- Method used to synchronise the cameras with each other (and with other data acquisition systems if used);
- Details of lighting (e.g. position of floodlights);
- Dimensions of 2D scaling object(s) or 3D performance volume (including number and location of control points).

Video digitising

- Digitising hardware and software (manufacturer and model/version);
- Resolution of the digitising system;
- Digitising rate (this may be less than the camera's frame rate);
- Model used (e.g. 15 point segmental).

Processing, analysing and reporting

- Algorithm used to obtain the 3D co-ordinates;
- Method used to smooth/filter the coordinates;
- Level of smoothing;
- Method used to obtain the derivative data (e.g. numerical, analytical);
- Source of segment inertia data used to calculate e.g. the whole body mass centre or moment of inertia;
- Definitions of the dependent variables being quantified, including their SI units;
- Estimation of the measurement error in the calculated parameters;
- Level of inter- and intra-observer reliability of the calculated parameters.

ACKNOWLEDGEMENT

I would like to thank Ed Parker for his help in preparing some of the photographs in this chapter and his technical advice. I would also like to thank Mark Johnson for providing high speed video footage for Figure 2.4.

REFERENCES

Abdel-Aziz, Y.I. and Karara, H.M. (1971) 'Direct linear transformation from comparator co-ordinates into object space co-ordinates in close range photogrammetry', in *American Society of Photogrammetry Symposium on Close Range Photogrammetry*, Falls Church, VA: American Society of Photogrammetry.

Andrews, J.G. (1995) 'Euler's and Lagrange's equations for linked rigid-body models of three-dimensional human motion', in P. Allard, I.A.F. Stokes and J-P. Blanchi (eds) *Three-dimensional analysis of human movement*, Champaign, IL: Human Kinetics.

Atkinson, G. and Nevill, A.M. (1998) 'Statistical methods for assessing measurement error (reliability) in variables relevant to sports medicine', *Sports Medicine*, 26(4): 217–238.

Bartlett, R.M. (1997a) *Introduction to Sports Biomechanics*, 1st edn, London: E & FN Spon.

Bartlett, R.M. (ed.) (1997b) *Biomechanical Analysis of Movement in Sport and Exercise*, Leeds: British Association of Sport and Exercise Sciences.

Brewin, M.A. and Kerwin, D.G. (2003) 'Accuracy of scaling and DLT reconstruction techniques for planar motion analyses', *Journal of Applied Biomechanics*, 19: 79–88.

Challis, J., Bartlett, R.M. and Yeadon, M. (1997) 'Image-based motion analysis', in R.M. Bartlett (ed.) *Biomechanical Analysis of Movement in Sport and Exercise*, Leeds: British Association of Sport and Exercise Sciences.

Chow, J.W. (1993) 'A panning videographic technique to obtain selected kinematic characteristics of the strides in sprint hurdling', *Journal of Applied Biomechanics*, 9: 149–159.

Gervais, P., Bedingfield, E.W., Wronko, C., Kollias, I., Marchiori, G., Kuntz, J., Way, N. and Kuiper, D. (1989) 'Kinematic measurement from panned cinematography', *Canadian Journal of Sports Sciences*, 14: 107–111.

Greaves, J.O.B. (1995) 'Instrumentation in video-based three-dimensional systems', in P. Allard, I.A.F. Stokes and J-P. Blanchi (eds) *Three-dimensional Analysis of Human Movement*, Champaign, IL: Human Kinetics.

Hay, J.G. and Reid, J.G. (1982) *The Anatomical and Mechanical Bases of Human Motion*, Englewood Cliffs, NJ: Prentice Hall.

Kerwin, D.G. (1995) 'Apex/Target high resolution video digitising system' in J. Watkins (ed.) *Proceedings of the Sports Biomechanics Section of the British Association of Sport and Exercise Sciences*, Leeds: British Association of Sport and Exercise Sciences.

Martin, T.P. and Pongrantz, M.B. (1974) 'Mathematical correction for photographic perspective error', *Research Quarterly*, 45: 318–323.

Miller, D.I. and Nelson, R.C. (1973) *Biomechanics of Sport: a Research Approach*. Philadelphia, PA: Lea & Febiger.

Miller, N.R., Shapiro, R. and McLaughlin, T.M. (1980) 'A technique for obtaining spatial kinematic parameters of segments of biomechanical systems from cinematographic data', *Journal of Biomechanics*, 13: 535–547.

Robertson, D.G.E. (2004) 'Body segment parameters', in D.G.E. Robertson, G.E. Caldwell, J. Hamill, G. Kamen and S.N. Whittlesey (eds) *Research Methods in Biomechanics*, Champaign, IL: Human Kinetics.

Sanders, R., Psycharakis, S., McCabe, C., Naemi, R., Connaboy, C., Li, S., Scott, G. and Spence, A. (2006) 'Analysis of swimming technique: State of the art: Applications and implications', *Portuguese Journal of Sport Sciences*, 6, supl. 2: 20–24.

Smith, G. (1975) 'Photographic analysis of movement', in D.W. Grieve, D.I. Miller, D. Mitchelson, J.P. Paul and A.J. Smith (eds) *Techniques for the Analysis of Human Movement*, London: Lepus Books.

Williams, A.M. and Ericsson, K.A. (2005) 'Some considerations when applying the expert performance approach in sport', *Human Movement Science*, 24: 283–307.

Winter, D.A. (1990) *Biomechanics and Motor Control of Human Movement*, 2nd edn, New York: Wiley.

Yanai, T., Hay, J.G. and Gerot, J.T. (1996) 'Three-dimensional videography of swimming with panning periscopes', *Journal of Biomechanics*, 29: 673–678.

Yeadon, M.R. (1989) 'A method for obtaining three-dimensional data on ski jumping using pan and tilt cameras', *International Journal of Sports Biomechanics*, 5: 238–247.

Yeadon, M.R. and King, M.A. (1999) 'A method for synchronising digitised video data', *Journal of Biomechanics*, 32: 983–986.

Yu, B., Koh, T.J. and Hay, J.G. (1993) 'A panning DLT procedure for three-dimensional videography', *Journal of Biomechanics*, 26: 741–751.

CHAPTER 3

MOTION ANALYSIS USING ON-LINE SYSTEMS

Clare E. Milner

INTRODUCTION

Biomechanics is about movement, and the objective measurement and recording of three-dimensional human movement is a keystone of the discipline. On-line motion analysis is an essential tool for the study of movement in sport and exercise. As with all tools, motion analysis systems need a skilled and knowledgeable operator to get the most from them. The mark of a good biomechanist is having not only the technical skills to operate a system successfully and collect high quality data, but also the scientific training to use the tools available to further our knowledge of human movement in sport and exercise. In sport and exercise biomechanics, research questions typically have an applied focus, with the aim of furthering our knowledge of elite sports performance or the reduction and prevention of injury. The flip-side of this focus is allowing ourselves to be led by technology, collecting huge amounts of data and trying to find relationships between the many variables involved afterwards, without any clear and logical rationale. In such 'data dredging', biomechanists are seduced by the advanced technology at their disposal, at the expense of scientific rigour.

On-line motion analysis in sport and exercise is currently being applied to research questions relating to injury or performance in many sports. Many of these studies are investigating injury, trying to elucidate the mechanism of injury or identify the factors that put an individual at increased risk of sustaining an injury. This focus on injury isn't surprising when you consider that remaining injury-free is a fundamental precursor to remain in training and being able to compete successfully. Many research groups have studied running and running injuries, for several reasons, not least that running is a popular recreational exercise for many individuals, not just an elite competitive sport. Running is also associated with a high risk of overuse injury, owing to its repetitiveness. Furthermore, the associations between mechanics and injury are subtle and complex, with little hard evidence of relationships between biomechanical characteristics of runners and injury occurrence being obtained in over 30 years of research. As technology has become more advanced and the research questions posed have become better defined, progress is being made. Many other sports are being investigated using on-line motion analysis, including rowing, cricket, baseball and golf.

The aim of this chapter is to introduce the key issues that must be considered when designing a motion capture study, from equipment selection to reporting the finished study. There are various competing motion analysis systems on the market, but the basic principles of quality data collection remain constant. Once you have a project in development, and have considered the variables needed to answer your research questions, you will know which data you need to collect. This dictates your hardware and system requirements, which we will consider first. The next stage is designing a data collection protocol that will enable you to collect data efficiently, accurately and precisely. These data are then processed to produce the study variables, which must then be interpreted in relation to the research questions posed and presented in a clear way to illustrate the results of your study for others. Basic principles of good reporting in motion analysis will be considered in the final section.

By the end of this chapter you should be able to identify and address the main quality control issues in on-line motion analysis and have the knowledge to present and interpret the results of a study clearly and meaningfully. The chapters on Research Methods and Data Processing and Error Estimation provide the foundations of scientific knowledge to compliment the technical skills developed in this chapter.

EQUIPMENT CONSIDERATIONS

The right equipment is a fundamental consideration for the development of a successful project. Once the variables needed to answer your research question have been identified, you can determine your equipment requirements. In addition to these experimental requirements, several practical considerations must also be borne in mind.

Since all on-line motion analysis systems currently rely on some kind of marker tracking, the initial consideration must be what marker system is most appropriate for the movements that you will study. For example, hard-wired or active marker systems are only appropriate for movements that are contained within a small volume and do not involve multiple twists and turns. The permanent connection of these systems with their markers means that all marker positions are always identified, but may hinder the movement of the athlete. Most on-line motion analysis systems use passive markers to indicate the position and orientation of the body in three-dimensional space. These systems rely on the reflection of visible or infra red light by the highly reflective spherical markers. The reflections are detected by multiple cameras, which record the motion of the body.

A basic hardware consideration is the number of cameras required to track the markers attached to your participants successfully. This will be based on both the number of markers that are attached to the participant and the complexity of the movements being performed. Marker sets and camera positioning will be considered in the next section, but, basically, the greater the number of markers and the more complex the movement, the more cameras will be required to collect good quality data. Minimally, two cameras are needed to enable three-dimensional reconstruction of the location of a marker in space. However, this arrangement would severely restrict both the movements that could be performed and the placement of markers to enable them to be tracked successfully. Adding cameras improves marker tracking and enables more markers to be tracked, up to a point, by increasing the likelihood that at least two cameras will be able to see a marker at each sampling interval. Some camera redundancy is desirable, but as the number of cameras increases, other factors come into play, such as processing time and, in the real world, the cost of the system. The current recommendation from manufacturers is an eight camera system for sport and exercise biomechanics applications, although many research laboratories operate successfully with six cameras.

Commercially available hardware and software is evolving constantly and ever more advanced equipment is becoming available at less cost. Issues to consider when comparing systems or determining your laboratory's requirements include:

- type of system; for example, passive or active markers, magnetic tracking technology
- range of sampling frequencies
- number of cameras that can link to a system
- maximum camera resolution
- type of lighting provided; for example, visible or infra red
- type and range of lens options
- minimum useful marker size; for example, in a full body volume
- real time capability
- ability to synchronise other hardware and number of analogue channels available; for example, force plate, EMG
- calibration method; for example, cube or wand
- output file format; for example, c3d, ASCII or binary
- software availability; for example, gait analysis, research
- service and support options
- typical price: low, medium or high range

Manufacturers' websites are the best source of up to date information; a list of manufacturers and their websites is provided in Appendix 2.

DATA COLLECTION PROCEDURES

Hardware set-up

There are three key areas that need to be given thorough consideration during protocol development to ensure high quality data are collected: hardware set-up, calibration and marker sets. The stages in hardware set-up are the selection of appropriate camera settings, determination of the optimal capture volume and location of the most suitable camera positions for the chosen volume within the constraints of the laboratory space available.

Check camera lens settings

In general, the camera settings that are manipulated by the biomechanist are the f-stop and the focal length. These settings are specific to the size of lens being used and recommended settings for a particular system will be provided by the manufacturer. The f-stop is related to the amount of light allowed to pass through the lens, with a 'larger' f-stop (f-16 rather than f-2, for example) letting less light through the lens. Generally, the focal length is set to infinity to get the maximum depth of field from the camera view.

Determine the location and dimensions of the capture volume

The size of the capture volume is a key consideration, since it affects the resolution of the system and, therefore, the precision with which position data can be recorded. The chosen capture volume is a compromise between the need to accommodate the movement being studied and maximising the resolution of the system by using the smallest volume possible. The volume must be sufficiently large to accommodate the movement in question fully for all expected sizes of participant. It is important to remember that this may need to include, for example, the hand of an outstretched arm in throwing sports, not just the torso. However, the volume only needs to cover the portion of the movement that is being studied. For example, a complete running stride, from foot strike of one foot to the next foot strike of the same foot may be two metres long. However, if the research question relates only to the stance phase of running, the length of the capture volume in the direction of running could be reduced from around 2.5 m, which would be needed to ensure that a complete stride occurs within the volume, to around 1 m.

   Although it may appear simplest to use a large capture volume to ensure that no movement data are lost, this will adversely affect the resolution of the system, resulting in a loss of precision in your data. The field of view of each camera is composed of a fixed number of pixels, typically 640 rows by 480 columns, although high resolution camera systems have resolutions up to 2352 rows by 1728 columns of pixels. Regardless of the specific resolution, the field of view of the camera is represented by a fixed number of pixels. A pixel is the minimum precision to which a marker in the camera view can be located. If the chosen capture volume is large, each pixel represents a relatively larger part of the 'real world' than it would for a smaller capture volume. For example, if the width of the capture volume was 5 m, each of 640 pixels in the width of the camera view would represent 5000/640 mm or 7.8 mm of that width. However, if the width of the capture volume could be reduced to 1 m, each pixel would represent 1000/640 mm or 1.6 mm. Resolution is also affected by camera position in relation to the capture volume.

Place cameras appropriately around the chosen capture volume

In setting up a motion analysis laboratory, maximum flexibility in camera placement should be maintained. Wall-mounting of cameras is often used to keep the cameras out of harm's way and reduce the risk of them being knocked over or damaged during other laboratory activities. If cameras are to be wall-mounted, lighting arms provide some flexibility in camera position in all three planes. Depending on the size of the laboratory and the floor space available, this may be the most feasible option. Maximum flexibility is maintained by the use of camera tripods to position the cameras; however, these require a lot of floor space and are more vulnerable to accidental contact, which then requires at least the recalibration of the system and may knock the camera to the floor and damage it. Other camera mounting arrangements have included tracks around the walls of a laboratory, along which the cameras can be moved horizontally and vertically. The disadvantage of this arrangement is that the cameras cannot be brought any closer to the capture volume to maximise system resolution. A variation on the tripod method is the use of vertical posts mounted on the laboratory floor. These require considerably less floor space than tripods, but must be attached to the floor to remain upright and stable, reducing the flexibility of the set-up. In the typical motion analysis laboratory, which is used for multiple concurrent projects, the flexibility gained by the use of tripods is often preferable, as it enables cameras to be positioned around the most appropriately sized capture volume for each study.

Ensure 'dead space' in each camera's field of view is minimised

The most appropriate camera position is that which minimises the 'dead space' surrounding the chosen capture volume in the camera's field of view. Dead space is that part of the camera's field of view that will not contribute to the data collection because it lies outside the capture volume. The presence of dead space reduces the resolution of the system because it effectively reduces the number of pixels that are available to represent the capture volume. A small dead space is usually unavoidable, given the fixed aspect ratio of the camera view and the shape of the capture volume, particularly when the volume is viewed from a position that is not orthogonal to it. However, dead space in the camera view should be minimised by ensuring that the camera is close enough to the volume for its field of view to be filled by the volume. If your cameras have the traditional rectangular field of view, it may be necessary to rotate them through 90° to minimise the dead space around the capture volume. Most systems have an option that enables you to rotate the apparent view of the camera so that the image seen on the computer screen appears in its normal orientation, despite the rotation of the camera.

Typically, the cameras will be equally spaced around a cuboid capture volume. This arrangement maximises the separation between adjacent cameras and provides maximum coverage of the capture volume, reducing the likelihood of marker dropout, which happens when a marker is not seen by at least two cameras in a sample and, thus, its position cannot be reconstructed. In reality, laboratories are often not an ideal shape and camera position options may be further reduced by the presence of other equipment. Additionally, different sports may require unusually shaped capture volumes. For example, in studying a tennis serve, particularly if the path of the head of the racket is of interest, a very tall, but relatively narrow volume will be required to accommodate the height of an arm plus racket stretched overhead. A good starting point is still to space the cameras equally around the volume and then fine tune the individual positions to minimise dead space while ensuring that the entire volume can still be seen by the camera.

All of these hardware issues are inter-related. The choice of camera lens dictates how much of the laboratory space the field of view of the camera will see. In turn, this is related to the position of the camera in relation to the chosen capture volume to ensure that dead space is minimised. For example, a wide angle lens will need to be closer to the capture volume than a normal lens to reduce the dead space around the capture volume in the camera's field of view by a similar amount. Lens choice should reflect the experimental set-up.

Select an appropriate sampling rate for your set-up and experiment

Other considerations when setting up your system for data collection include the sampling rate or frequency and synchronisation with other equipment. In some cases, the sampling rate can be specified, with higher sampling rates being associated with decreased resolution in a trade-off associated with the processing power of the hardware. For example, cameras that have full resolution at 120 Hz (samples per second) may be able to capture data at 240 Hz, but only at 50 per cent of the spatial resolution. That is, there is a trade-off between temporal resolution and spatial resolution. Again, the most appropriate option for your study should be selected. If the capture volume is small, the loss of spatial resolution may be acceptable to allow a higher temporal resolution to capture a high-speed movement. The loss of spatial resolution associated with a large capture volume may be unacceptable and a lower temporal resolution must be chosen. Most human movements have a relatively low frequency, but where high speeds of movement and rapid changes of direction are involved, movement information may be lost if the sampling frequency is too low.

Synchronise other hardware at an appropriate sampling frequency

Most motion analysis systems can be synchronised with other biomechanical hardware through a series of analog input channels. This allows force platform, EMG or other analogue data to be time-synchronised with the kinematic data collection of the motion capture system. Other hardware typically samples at a higher frequency than the motion capture system. To enable the data sets to be time-synchronised, the higher frequency should be a multiple of the motion capture frequency.

Calibration

Calibrating the motion capture system enables the image coordinates on each individual camera view to be converted to the real world three-dimensional coordinates of each marker. For most systems this is a two-stage process with an initial static, or seed, calibration followed by a dynamic, or wand, calibration.

Determine the origin and orientation of the laboratory-fixed global axes

The static calibration uses a rigid L-frame with four markers mounted in known locations (Figure 3.1). The L-frame defines the location of the origin and the orientation of the laboratory reference frame. The orientation of the laboratory reference frame has no effect on the joint angles calculated from the three-dimensional coordinate data, but standard definitions have been suggested to make communication between laboratories easier. The International Society of Biomechanics (ISB) has suggested aligning the X axis with the direction of progression, the Y axis vertically and the Z axis mediolaterally to create a right-handed orthogonal coordinate system (Wu and Cavanagh, 1995). This orientation was suggested as it is a simple extension from sagittal plane two-dimensional analyses that have X oriented horizontally and Y vertically. Extension into the third dimension simply requires the addition of a mediolateral axis, the Z axis. A typical engineering definition of the laboratory coordinate system places X in the direction of progression, Y mediolateral and Z vertical. It should be noted that the Z axis in the ISB definition is equivalent to −Y in the engineering version, as both follow the right-hand rule.

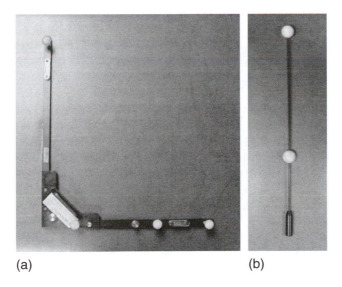

(a)   (b)

Figure 3.1   (a) The L-frame used in the static calibration of a motion capture system and its relationship to the laboratory reference frame; (b) The wand used in the dynamic calibration

Determine an acceptable residual for your set-up

A good calibration is fundamental to the collection of high quality data. The position of the markers in three-dimensional space can only be located to the accuracy to which the system was calibrated. At the end of the calibration process, the data capture software typically provides an indication of the precision that can be achieved based on the calibration done. Each camera has a residual associated with it. This number, in the units in which the system was calibrated, provides an indication of the precision to which the marker position can be located. For example, a residual of 1.0 mm indicates that a marker's position in space will be located to within 1 mm of its true position. Larger capture volumes will have higher residuals for the same quality of calibration owing to the resolution of the system being based on a fixed number of pixels in each camera view (see Hardware set-up section above).

Adjust camera sensitivity

The static calibration is the first stage of the two-stage calibration process. It is important to place the L-frame in the correct orientation with respect to the laboratory, and any additional hardware such as force platforms, if the global axes are to be used as a reference for any of your variables, for example toe-out angle during running. For this part of the calibration to succeed, camera sensitivity must be checked. The camera sensitivity changes the intensity at which the camera will register a reflection and try to reconstruct it as a marker. If the sensitivity is set too high, lots of stray reflections will be picked up in addition to those from the actual markers. If too low, the markers themselves will not be recognised.

Check for stray reflections in each camera's field of view

When the sensitivity of each camera has been adjusted, the individual camera views should be checked for additional reflective objects, for example, other cameras. Some software enables those parts of the camera view that contain an unwanted object to be blocked out, but this part of the view is also blocked during data collection. It is good practice, and a necessity for some types of software, to ensure that camera views are adjusted to avoid stray reflections being picked up. If a reflection is picked up by more than one camera, it will be reconstructed as a marker and the static calibration will fail.

Perform static calibration

The only markers that can be present in the camera views during calibration are those on the L-frame.

Perform dynamic calibration

After a successful static calibration, the dynamic calibration is conducted to register the cameras to the whole of the capture volume. The wand calibration is basically the direct measurement of an object of known dimensions made by all the cameras throughout the entire capture volume. Each system manufacturer has its preferred style of wand calibration, but the fundamental requirements are that the whole volume is covered and that the orientation of the wand is varied to ensure accurate calibration in all three cardinal planes.

Ensure a valid calibration is maintained throughout the data collection session

Calibration should be done before every data collection session, even if the cameras are wall-mounted and do not appear to move between sessions. Calibration is a sensitive procedure and even a small vibration of a camera can move it sufficiently to reduce the quality of the reconstruction of marker location. If a camera is knocked or moved during a data collection session, the system should be recalibrated. Every effort should be taken to avoid this, such as asking participants to take care not to touch the cameras and having as few people as possible moving about the laboratory during data collection. However, the calibration procedure is easy and takes only a few minutes. If in doubt, it is always worth recalibrating to be sure that you are maintaining the quality of your data. A good indicator that the quality of your calibration has been reduced is the appearance of ghost markers in your capture volume. Ghost markers are markers that are reconstructed by the software based on the information from the cameras and the calibration parameters, but that do not actually exist. Other reasons to recalibrate include changing the units of measurement or the orientation of the laboratory coordinate system, although in practice these changes would be unlikely to occur during a data collection session.

Marker sets

A marker set is simply a configuration of markers that meets the selection criteria defined by Cappozzo *et al.*, 1995.

A minimum of three non-collinear markers is required per rigid segment for three-dimensional analysis

Three non-collinear markers are required on a segment to define its position and orientation in three-dimensional space. Two markers define a line and can provide information about two-dimensional movement but cannot indicate whether rotation about that line is occurring. A third non-collinear marker, which does not lie on the line, is needed to define this axial rotation of the segment.

Each marker must be seen by at least two cameras at every instant during data recording

This is the minimum requirement for three-dimensional reconstruction of the marker position in three-dimensional space, although reconstruction accuracy may be improved when some redundancy is introduced and more cameras can see the markers. Furthermore, the inter-marker distances must be sufficient that the system can differentiate between individual markers during marker reconstruction. If markers are placed too close together, the system will be unable to identify where one marker begins and the other ends. In this case, only one marker will be reconstructed instead of the two. Additionally, the further apart a segment markers can be placed, the smaller the impact of marker position reconstruction error on the joint angles that are calculated from the raw coordinate data.

Minimise movement between the markers and the underlying bone

The aim of on-line motion analysis is to determine the movement of the underlying bone structures by recording the movement of markers mounted on the skin's surface. The discrepancy between the movement of the marker and the actual movement of the skeleton is known as 'skin movement artefact'. The gold standard for marker mounting is to attach markers directly to the bones of interest using bone pins. Although this has been done in a few studies, it is obviously impractical in most cases as it is invasive. However, comparison studies between bone pin and skin-mounted markers provide an indication of the magnitude and type of error associated with skin-marker measurement. There are two types of skin-marker movement error, absolute and relative (Nigg and Herzog, 1999). Errors due to skin-marker movement at the knee during walking may be up to 10 per cent of the flexion–extension range of motion, 50 per cent of the abduction–adduction range of motion and 100 per cent of the internal–external rotation range of motion (Cappozzo *et al.*, 1996). Minimising skin movement artefact must be the main criterion in marker set design (Cappozzo *et al.*, 1996).

Marker set selection and development

Determine the type of marker set that is most appropriate for your study

The choice of an appropriate marker set is critical to ensuring that all of your required variables can be calculated from the raw data collected. It also plays a key role in the quality of your data set, related to skin movement artefact and the introduction of noise into the data. Choosing an appropriate marker set and mounting it accurately on the skin is essential to obtaining data that are representative of the movement being studied. There are three main options when determining the marker set to use in your study (Figure 3.2). The first is

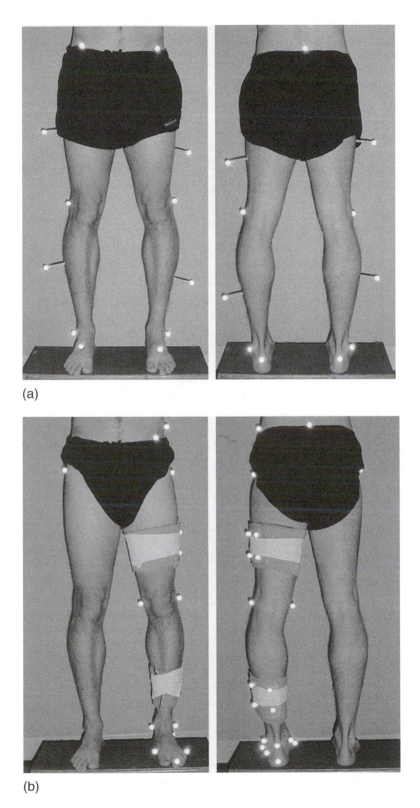

(a)

(b)

Figure 3.2 Marker sets used in on-line motion analysis: (a) Standard clinical gait analysis marker set; (b) Cluster-based marker set

to use one of the standard clinical gait analysis marker sets to answer your question. Alternatively, you can design your own marker set with markers attached to anatomical points of your choice. Finally, you could use markers attached to rigid thermoplastic clusters that are then attached to the participant. Each of these methods has advantages and disadvantages.

Use the standard clinical gait analysis marker set

The advantages of the standard clinical gait analysis marker set are that it has been tried and tested in many laboratories throughout the world and has been used in very many studies over the past 20 years. The main manufacturers also provide software that will automatically process raw data obtained using this marker set through to time-normalised mean graphs for each variable. However, this marker set has several serious limitations, related to the small number of markers used. The most serious limitations are at the foot, which has only two markers on it. Consequently, the multi-segmented foot is represented simply as a line, making true three-dimensional rotation information about this segment, relative to the leg, impossible. Additionally, the shank has only two markers on it (the only marker at the knee joint is located on the femoral condyle). Furthermore, since this marker set was designed originally for lower extremity gait analysis during walking, applying it to sports movements may not be valid and may reduce its effectiveness, both in terms of markers being obscured from camera views and also in minimising marker movement. For example, the placement of markers on wands to improve the estimation of transverse plane rotations may result in unacceptably high marker vibration at impact during higher speed activities. However, this source of error can easily be reduced by placing these markers directly on the skin.

Design a custom marker set

An alternative is to design a custom marker set for your study that follows the rule of three markers per rigid segment; necessary for true three-dimensional motion capture. This enables some of the limitations highlighted above to be overcome. However, a good knowledge of surface anatomy is needed to determine the most appropriate marker locations that both minimise skin movement artefact and enable joint centres to be located. Typically, two markers are needed to define the relative location of a joint centre and the third marker is placed somewhere in the middle of the segment away from the line between the two anatomical markers to enable the three-dimensional position and orientation of the segment to be recorded. Additional markers may be placed on a segment to ensure that at least three are visible in every frame of data collected. This is a consideration for complex sports movements that involved twisting and bending of the body that may obscure certain markers.

Develop and use a cluster-based marker set

The third option is the use of marker clusters that are placed on the middle region of the segment and have a known relationship to the anatomical points required for data processing. This method allows more flexibility in camera placement as the clusters can be positioned on the segment in the orientation that makes them most visible to the cameras. This is particularly useful if only a few cameras are available or the laboratory environment restricts camera placement options. However, this method necessitates an extra step – the collection of a static trial. Static trials are often used with the other types of markers set to provide a zero reference position for joint angles and to define joint centre locations using markers on different segments. However, with marker clusters one or a series of static trials is required to locate the anatomical points relative to the cluster. If a single static trial is used, markers are placed on all of the anatomical points and their relationships to the cluster calculated during data processing. An alternative method (Cappozzo *et al.*, 1995) uses a pointer to locate each anatomical point. This method requires a separate static trial for each anatomical point, but does not require that all of the anatomical markers are visible simultaneously, unlike the single trial method. Therefore, it can be used in those setups that have restricted camera placement options.

Introduce asymmetry into your marker set to optimise marker tracking

Asymmetry can be introduced in your marker set simply by adding an additional marker to one side of the body. Additionally, non-anatomical markers on each segment can be varied in placement between the right and left sides. The asymmetry enables the software algorithms, which use the distances and angles between markers to identify them, to work more effectively.

Consider marker size

Marker size is a compromise between having a marker large enough to be seen by several cameras and to cover multiple pixels, which improves the accuracy of the location of its position, but not so large that it interferes with movement of the athlete or overlaps with other markers in the camera view. The standard clinical gait analysis marker set uses 25 mm markers, but high-resolution cameras can be used successfully with 5 mm markers.

Use an appropriate method of marker attachment

Mounting the markers on the skin must be fast and easy and the attachment must remain secure for the duration of data collection. Various methods are used for marker attachment. Marker attachment directly on the skin is preferable. Markers attached to clothing have another layer between them and the bone, introducing the possibility of further movement artefact. Double-sided tape, such as toupee tape and electrocardiography (ECG) discs are used to attach the markers. If these are insufficient, adhesive sprays may be used to provide additional adhesion, for example if the participant will sweat during the data collection. In some instances tight-fitting Lycra clothing is used and markers are attached using Velcro. This method is quick and avoids any discomfort for the participant associated with pulling adhesive tape off the skin, but introduces the extra layer of movement between the marker and the bone.

Take great care with marker placement

It must also be emphasised that the marker set is only as good as the person who applies it to the participant. If the markers used in the determination of joint centre locations are misplaced relative to the underlying bony anatomy, the joint centres used in data processing and analysis will not be coincident with the actual joint centres, so cross-talk will be introduced into the kinematic data. Consistent marker placement between investigators and between days is notoriously difficult to achieve. It is recommended that only one person places markers on all participants in a study to remove inter-individual variability as a source of error.

PROCESSING, ANALYSING AND PRESENTING MOTION ANALYSIS DATA

Data processing

The first stage in data processing is cleaning the data, which means checking that the markers are identified correctly in every frame, joining any broken trajectories and deleting unnamed markers. Current on-line motion capture software removes the need for manual identification of markers in each frame of data collected. In the past, this onerous task was the rate-limiting factor in processing human movement data. Nowadays, marker identification either occurs in real-time or takes place in a matter of seconds after data collection. However, the software is not fool proof and each trial collected must be checked to ensure that markers have been identified correctly. This is simple pattern recognition as the template used to join the markers can be recognised and deviation from the correct template can be readily seen by eye. The additional work needed at this stage can be minimised by designing a robust marker set, with planned asymmetries, and an associated template before data collection.

Secondly, if a good camera set-up and appropriate choice of marker set is made initially, the number of broken trajectories and size of the breaks should be minimal. There are two schools of thought on joining broken trajectories. One is that any line joining is unacceptable and the hardware set-up should be refined and new trials recorded until complete trajectories are obtained. The other is that small breaks in marker trajectories that are not at peaks or changes in direction of the curve are acceptable for around five consecutive data samples. Most software offers quintic spline curve-fitting techniques, which adequately reproduce the curve provided that the curve is only undergoing minor changes during the period when data are missing. This makes practical sense in that whole trials do not need to be rejected as a result of a minor dropout of a single marker for a few samples, but data are rejected if multiple markers are lost or the period of marker dropout is significant.

Thirdly, unnamed markers need to be deleted from the trial before the data is processed. These unnamed markers are the ghost markers referred to earlier and do not contribute any information about the movement of the participant. Before deleting these markers, you should make sure that all of the body markers are identified correctly and none has been switched with a ghost marker by the template recognition algorithm of the software. Additionally, you should ensure that apparently broken trajectories are not simply points where the algorithm has failed to recognise a body marker and it has become temporarily unnamed. When you are satisfied that any unnamed markers are, indeed, ghost markers they should be deleted from the trial so that the data processing software functions properly.

Filtering is another important consideration with human movement data. Since it is covered in detail elsewhere in this book, only basic considerations will be raised here. Noise due to skin marker movement is generally of high frequency and human movement occurs at low frequencies; therefore, the two can be separated using a low-pass filter. Such a filter separates the components of the time-displacement curve of a marker based on whether the components oscillate above or below a chosen cut-off frequency, and discards all components above the cut-off. The cut-off frequency used can have a significant effect on the shape of the marker trajectory: too low and the curve becomes over-smoothed – the peaks are flattened; too high and the curve remains noisy. Cut-off frequencies can be determined using specific algorithms, plotting a frequency distribution curve or by trial and error sampling of different cut-off frequencies and observing their effect on the data. As an indication of cut-off frequencies used for different movements, walking data are typically filtered at 6 Hz, running at 8 Hz to 12 Hz.

Once the raw data have been prepared in this way, they can be analysed to obtain the kinematic variables needed to answer your research question.

Data analysis

The methods of data analysis used in your study depend on the type of system you have and the marker set that you used. If you use the standard gait analysis marker set, most systems provide software that processes the raw data automatically and provides plots of all the variables as output. This method is simple to use, but does not give the biomechanist any control over the calculation methods. If you choose to use a custom marker set you may be able to use the research software provided by the system manufacturer. This allows you to define the segment coordinate systems and other components of your data analysis from options written into the software. This additional flexibility provides more control over the data analysis stage of your study, but relies on your technical knowledge being sufficient to make the correct decisions about segment coordinate axis definitions, joint coordinate system calculations and orders of rotation. For complete control over the data analysis process, the final option is to write your own software using a computer or engineering programming language. With this method you can be confident that all of the calculations are exactly as you intend and you have complete flexibility in your choice of data collection method. However, writing and validating such code for three-dimensional kinematic analysis is a major task requiring excellent technical and mathematical knowledge and a significant time commitment: it should not be undertaken lightly.

Regardless of the method chosen, the end result of data analysis is the extraction of three-dimensional kinematic data from the raw marker position data collected during the movement trials. The basic output is angular variables, or their derivatives, against time for each trial. These data may then be further manipulated or reduced to aid data interpretation.

Data interpretation and presentation

There are many options for interpreting and presenting motion analysis data. To aid the interpretation of reduced data – discrete values such as peaks – it is useful to present time-normalised mean curves to enable qualitative interpretation of the data. It should always be remembered that the average curve smoothes the peaks of the individual trials as a result of inter-trial temporal differences. The most appropriate way of presenting these data will depend on your project, and the variability between trials (Figure 3.3). If all trials are very similar, a single mean curve may be most appropriate. However, an indication of the variability between trials is usually helpful, and a mean ± 1 standard deviation curves will often be more informative. In other cases, it may be better to plot all of the individual curves on the same graph, to give the reader all of the information about inter-trial variability. Mean values for the key variables are reported alongside these plots.

Data reduction means extracting key variables from the continuous data obtained during data processing. Typical variables are peaks of angular displacement or velocity, or angles at defined instants. For example, peak rear-foot eversion and inversion angle at foot strike are discrete variables that are often considered in research questions about running injuries. The key decision to make when reducing data is whether to extract the discrete data points from the time-normalised mean curve, or from the individual trial curves and then calculate a mean value for the variable in question. For times that are clearly defined by an event in the time domain, the output will be the same. For example, rear-foot angle at foot-strike is unaffected because it defines the same data point on each individual curve as on the mean curve. However, extracting data from the individual curves is more appropriate for peak values because it preserves the time domain variability information. The mean curve tends to reduce the apparent peak values when they occur at different times.

Depending on the research question asked, other types of analysis may be appropriate. For example, much current research is concerned with the coordination between segments and how coordination variability may affect injury risk. A detailed review of techniques used to quantify and assess variability is beyond the scope of this chapter.

The common thread in current analyses of human movement data is the extraction of discrete variables from continuous time-series data. The discrete variables are used to answer your research questions statistically. To maintain the statistical power of your study, it is preferable to identify a few key variables

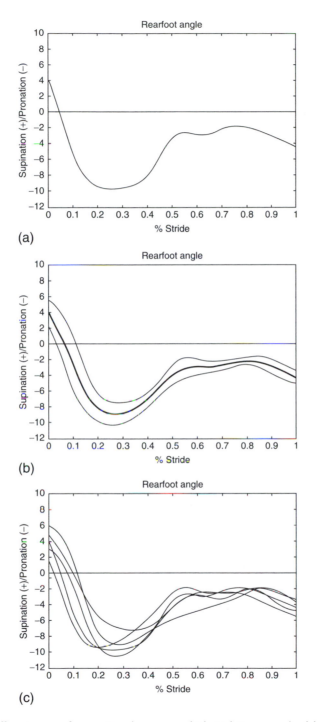

Figure 3.3 Different ways of presenting the same multiple-trial time-normalised kinematic data: (a) mean curve; (b) mean ± 1 standard deviation curves; (c) all individual curves. The example shown is rear-foot motion during running

that will contribute the most to your hypotheses and present other associated variables, continuous and discrete, descriptively to aid in the interpretation of your statistical results.

REPORTING A MOTION ANALYSIS STUDY

This section contains general guidelines for reporting a motion capture study. The detail required in specific sections will vary depending on the purpose of the report: whether it is a report to a research group or commissioned research for a consultancy client. For example, the client that commissioned a piece of research may only be interested in broadbrush detail of your methods, but may require in depth explanation of your results in non-technical layman's terms.

Introduction

- Introduce the general area in broad terms.
- Focus on the specific topic of your study.
- Describe the current state of knowledge briefly by referring to existing literature.
- Highlight the gap in the literature that your study addresses.
- End with a statement of your aims and hypotheses.

Methods

- Begin with participant demographics, including only those that are relevant to interpretation of the study or were used in participant selection.
- Follow with statements about ethics board approval and participant written informed consent.
- Include sufficient detail of experimental procedure for a knowledgeable biomechanist to reproduce your study exactly.
- Do not reproduce the detail of standard procedures, but provide a primary reference that contains full details, should the reader be unfamiliar with the procedures.
- If appropriate, include a section on statistical analysis that contains details of the tests used and the dependent and independent variables used to test your hypotheses.

Results

- Part of the skill of a biomechanical investigator is to be able to tease out those data that are relevant to their research questions and use these to construct a focused and informative results section.

- Include only those data that address the aims of your study. Including every result that your data processing software spilled out does not impress the reader with how much work you did. Instead, it forces them to conclude that you did not know what question your study was trying to answer.

- The results section should contain details of the variables that were tested statistically, and the results of the statistical tests done. It helps the reader to interpret your results if the actual P values obtained are reported, rather than whether or not a particular level of significance was reached.

- Descriptive statistics of those secondary variables that were not related directly to your hypotheses, but aid in the interpretation of the primary variables, should also be included.

- Figures and tables should be included as necessary for clarity, but should not replicate the same information.

- Text in this section should summarise the results and draw attention to relevant details contained within figures and tables.

- Remember that the purpose of this section is to present the results of your study: their interpretation occurs in the Discussion section.

Discussion

- The results presented are interpreted with reference to the literature that was included in the Introduction.

- Do not introduce new concepts or literature in this section. The Discussion ties together all of the information that has been presented in the Introduction, Methods and Results sections. Any existing literature that you want to refer to should be included in your Introduction and any results you want to discuss should be contained within the Results section.

- Comment on whether your initial hypotheses were supported or rejected by the results obtained and discuss the implications of this.

- Summarise what has been learned from your study and draw conclusions about your research questions, if this is appropriate.

- Be careful not to make grand sweeping statements based on your study. Increasing knowledge and understanding of a biomechanical problem is a stepwise process. Acknowledge the contribution your study makes, but avoid extrapolating beyond its parameters.

- Be sure to acknowledge any limitations of your study and how these might affect the interpretation of your results.

- Discuss whether the aims of the study set out in the Introduction have been achieved and, if not, comment on why not and what might be done in the future to address this.

- If the study is part of a bigger picture, it may be appropriate to refer to future plans to build on the knowledge gained and address further relevant questions in the research topic.

References

- Include a complete list of all the literature that has been referred to in the body of your report. It is important that the list is accurate to enable the reader to follow up on aspects that are of particular interest.
- Literature that you want to highlight to the reader that has not been referred to directly in the report should be put in a bibliography at the end of the report. Note that a bibliography is not usually included in scientific reports, but may be useful in a report to a consultancy client to enable them to learn more about specific areas.

The most important consideration when compiling your report is that it follows a logical order, from the development of a research question through data that relates to that question and, finally, ties together existing knowledge and new results from your study to answer the research question and add another piece of understanding to the puzzle of human movement in sport and exercise.

Having reached the end of this chapter, you should now be familiar with all of the main quality control and technical issues related to on-line motion analysis as a data collection tool in sport and exercise biomechanics. Every project is different and has specific requirements and pitfalls. Preparation is the key to success and time spent addressing the issues raised at the outset of the study will help to prevent problems later, after the participants have made their contributions.

ACKNOWLEDGEMENT

I would like to thank John D. Willson for kindly agreeing to act as the model for Figure 3.2.

REFERENCES

Cappozzo, A., Catini, F., Della Croce, U. and Leardini, A. (1995) 'Position and orientation in space of bones during movement: anatomical frame definition and determination', *Clinical Biomechanics*, 10: 171–178.

Cappozzo, A., Catini, F., Leardini, A., Benedetti, M.G. and Della Croce, U. (1996) 'Position and orientation in space of bones during movement: experimental artefacts', *Clinical Biomechanics*, 11: 90–100.

Nigg, B.M. and Herzog, W. (eds) (1999) *Biomechanics of the Musculo-skeletal System*, Chichester, UK: Wiley & Sons Ltd.

Wu, G. and Cavanagh, P.R. (1995) 'ISB recommendations for standardization in the reporting of kinematic data', *Journal of Biomechanics*, 28: 1257–1261.

CHAPTER 4

FORCE AND PRESSURE MEASUREMENT

Adrian Lees and Mark Lake

INTRODUCTION

The force of contact between the human and the environment, and the associated localised forces or pressures produced over small areas of this contact, are fundamental to our understanding of how humans perform in a sport or exercise context. Knowledge about the forces and pressures acting during an activity enables us to understand more about the general way that humans use their body and limbs to achieve desired outcomes and more detail about how these forces are generated and the effect that these forces have on and within the body. Thus, knowledge of forces and pressures helps us to understand more about performance and injury mechanisms.

This chapter is concerned with the theoretical and practical aspects of the tools used to measure and evaluate forces and pressures in sport and exercise biomechanics. Because there are many such systems available, the focus will be on the major systems. Thus, for force measurement this chapter will focus on the force platform while for pressure measurement it will focus on systems used to measure plantar pressures on the foot.

THE FORCE PLATFORM

Background and brief history

The way humans mechanically operate in sport and exercise situations is due to the interaction of a number of forces. Some of these forces are produced internally to the body, such as muscle force, while others are produced by nature, such as gravity and air resistance, yet others still are produced by the interaction that we have with our environment, such as contact forces. A typical

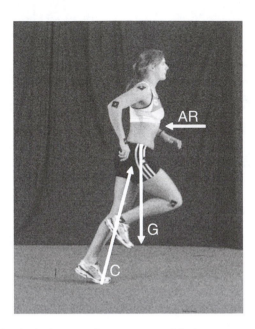

Figure 4.1 Force (or free body diagram) illustrating some of the forces (contact, C, gravity, G and air resistance, AR) acting on the runner

force (or free body) diagram for an athlete is given in Figure 4.1. Many of the external forces such as gravity and air resistance can be estimated from mathematical formulae worked out over the centuries. However, the contact forces cannot easily be estimated in this way and so it is necessary to measure them. These contact forces can then be used as direct representations of a movement or used in analytical formulae (such as the equations of motion based on Newton's Second law) in order to perform a full mechanical analysis of a situation.

Because the measurement of force is so important to a further understanding of the way we operate, force measuring devices have been developed. These devices have traditionally been force platforms located in the ground, due to the importance of the foot–ground interface in both sport and exercise situations. They can of course also be located on a wall or within other apparatus, for example, a diving platform.

The first force measuring device used in human motion is usually attributed to Marey, the French Physiologist, in 1895 (see Nigg and Herzog, 1994). This system used air-filled tubes, which could register the pressure – and hence force – of the foot on the ground. This elaborate equipment, carried by the runner himself, had many shortcomings and subsequent investigators preferred to have the measuring device separate from the participant. Force sensitive platforms were built to react to both vertical and horizontal forces. One example, the 'trottoir dynamographique' of Amar in 1916 (see Cavanagh, 1990) reacted by means of rubber bulbs that were compressed by the movement of the platform. In 1938 Elftman built a platform that used springs to register the forward or backward forces of a runner's foot against the ground (see Nigg and Herzog, 1994). The limitation of this apparatus was the displacement necessary to compress the springs and the low natural frequency of the platform itself.

Subsequently, more sophisticated designs became available based on rigid supports that were strain gauged or composed of piezo-electric material (see Nigg and Herzog, 1994 for a detailed explanation of these measuring methods). This enabled the platform to become effectively non-deformable (although minute oscillations still occurred) and to have a high natural frequency so that impacts could be faithfully recorded.

The first commercial force platform was manufactured by Kistler in 1969 and used the piezo-electric principle; it quickly became accepted as a world standard for force measurement. In 1976 Advanced Mechanical Technology Incorporated (AMTI, USA) introduced a strain gauge platform which had the advantages of a larger surface area and lower price. These two commercial force platforms still remain the most popular force platforms world wide, although others have subsequently become commercially available.

Construction and operation

Commercial force platforms are rectangular in shape and available in a variety of sizes and constructional types. A typical example is the Kistler 9281B force platform, which is a solid metal base plate, has dimensions of $600 \times 400 \times 60$ mm and weighs 410 N. It can measure forces ranging from 10–10,000 N and is accurate to two per cent of the measuring range used. The platform has a high natural frequency (>200 Hz) and has good linearity in measurement.

The typical force platform can measure six variables which have their positive sense as shown in Figure 4.2. This axis system represents the forces acting *on* the body and these are strictly termed reaction forces. Thus, the action force applied to the ground when contact is made causes a reaction force which acts on the body (Newton's Third law tells us that these must be equal and opposite). It makes sense to deal with the forces as they act on the body as

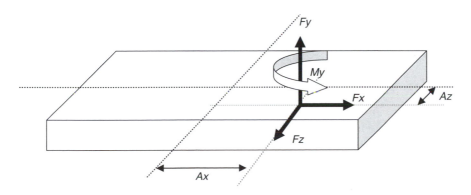

Figure 4.2   The force platform measurement variables

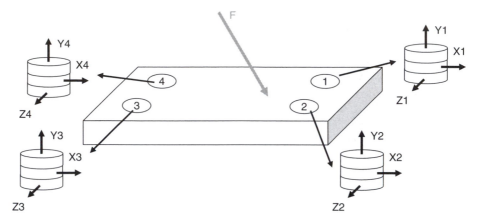

Figure 4.3   The three component load cells embedded at each corner of the force platform

these are used for any biomechanical analysis, as illustrated in Figure 4.1. The six variables are:

> Fx, Fy and Fz – the reaction forces along the respective co-ordinate axes;
> Ax and Az – the co-ordinates which identify the point of force application or centre of pressure and
> My – the friction torque (or free moment) about the vertical axis.

The platform has a load cell in each of its four corners (Figure 4.3). Each load cell is constructed so that it is sensitive to forces along each of the X, Y or Z axes (the actual construction of the load cell depends on whether it uses the piezo-electric or strain gauge principle). The principle of operation is that when an external force F is applied, a reaction force is generated by the load cells to retain equilibrium (i.e. $\Sigma F = 0$).

A total of 12 individual reaction forces are produced by the three components of each of the four load cells. Applying standard mechanical analysis to these forces we can compute the resultant component reaction forces (Fx, Fy and Fz) as follows:

$$Fx = X1 + X2 + X3 + X4 \tag{4.1}$$
$$Fy = Y1 + Y2 + Y3 + Y4 \tag{4.2}$$
$$Fz = Z1 + Z2 + Z3 + Z4 \tag{4.3}$$

Obtaining the other three measurements (Ax, Az and My) is a little more difficult and you should refer to the manufacturer's technical manual or Nigg and Herzog, 1994, for further detail. Suffice to say these variables are obtained from the same 12 load cell values and can be given as:

$$Ax = (Y1 + Y2 - Y3 - Y4)b/Fy \tag{4.4}$$
$$Az = (Y1 + Y4 - Y2 - Y3)a/Fy \tag{4.5}$$
$$My = (X1 + X2 - X3 - X4)a + (Z1 + Z4 - Z2 - Z3)b \tag{4.6}$$

Where Fy is given by equation 4.2, and the dimensions 'a' and 'b' refer to the distance of the load cells from the centre of the platform in the Z and X directions, respectively.

There are three important issues that need to be addressed at this stage:

1   The identity of the axes used to define each direction varies in the literature. In the preferred system (as recommended by the International Society of Biomechanics) the vertical axis is Y, although some force platform manufacturers, and many published papers, designate the vertical axis as Z. The choice of axes' names is largely historical and is an unnecessary source of confusion, but as this situation is unlikely to change we need to be aware of the different axes identities used.

2   Strictly the force platform measures the forces acting on it (the action force) so we need to take into account the action–reaction principle to establish the forces acting on the person. When a force is applied to the force platform the load cells record this action force, but the force which acts on the person is the equal and opposite reaction to this. Thus, a downward (negative lab axis direction) force acting on the platform is recorded as an upward (positive) force representing the reaction force acting on the body. This same principle also applies to the horizontal forces and free moment, and in order to achieve a suitable right hand co-ordinate system representing the forces acting on the person, some adjustment to signs needs to be made. These are usually incorporated within the analysis software and are not apparent to the user but a check should always be made to ensure the correct sense of direction is known for each force platform variable. This is easily done by running over the platform in different directions, noting the directions of the resulting force curves, and comparing these to typical curves for running (e.g. Figure 4.4 in Interpretation of Force Variables section).

3   The analysis leading to equations 4.4, 4.5 and 4.6 assumes that the external force is applied to the force platform in the same horizontal plane as measured by the load cells. In most cases this is not the case and certainly will not be if an artificial surface is applied to the force platform. Under these conditions a correction needs to be made to these equations. These will usually be incorporated within any analysis software and will also be detailed in the manufacturer's technical specification.

Technical specification

The force platform system comprises a number of hardware items (transducer – the platform itself, signal conditioning device and signal recording device) and software for signal processing. Each item is considered here in turn.

The force platform together with the signal conditioning hardware should result in good linearity, low hysteresis, good range of measurement, appropriate sensitivity, low cross-talk and excellent dynamic response. Typical values are:

Range	axes: vertical $-10 - +20$ kN ; horizontal ± 10 kN
Linearity	<0.5% full scale deflection
Hysteresis	<0.5% full scale deflection
Cross-talk	<2%
Natural frequency	high >700 Hz in vertical axis
Temperature range	-20 to $+ 50$ C

The reader is referred to Bartlett, 1997, for more detailed information on each of these items. Modern commercial force platforms have, through a process of development in transducer and signal conditioning electronics, managed to achieve these performance requirements. While there are differences between platforms due to transducer type, construction and size (and the purchaser and user should make themselves aware of these) in general, modern commercial force platform systems are suitable for purpose. A note should be added here on installation. This would normally have been done according to the manufacturer's instructions, which specify the inclusion of an inertial mass, isolation from the immediate building surroundings and location on a non-suspended (i.e. ground) floor. Some force platform locations, through necessity, do not conform to these requirements and artefacts may be noticeable in the data. The user should satisfy themselves of the conditions of installation, and be aware of potential problems, particularly with impacts and rapidly changing force levels.

Signal recording is nowadays almost exclusively undertaken by computer which is linked to the hardware device for analogue-to-digital (AD) conversion. The signal representing the force platform variables is available from the system's amplifier as an analogue voltage; usually within the range of ± 10 V. The analogue signal is converted to digital data by an AD converter, which would normally be a 12 or 16-bit device. For a 12-bit device the signal is converted to 2^{12} (4096) levels. This is quite adequate for force measurement as it means that a signal within the range of ± 5000 N (typical for most sports activities) can be resolved to 2.4 N. This is better than the inherent noise within the signal, which can be seen if a base line measurement is amplified to cover a 10 N range. For activities in which the forces are lower, for example gait analysis with children, a lower measuring range may be selected so that the sensitivity of the recording may be as low as 1 N. A 16-bit AD converter would provide a sensitivity of recording far in excess of that required for all types of measurement.

Signal processing is performed by proprietary software supplied by the manufacturer or by custom written software available within a laboratory setting. Most users will only be aware of the final six force platform variables. However, writing custom software is not problematic if you have appropriate skills and the availability of some high level package such as Matlab, Labview or even Excel, and may be an interesting exercise at postgraduate level. In either case the 'raw' signals from the platform's load cells need to be processed in order to derive the force platform variables using equations similar to equations 4.1–4.6. The specific equations required are system dependent so you will need to refer to the manufacturer's technical specification for this. In implementing these equations, account must be taken of the sense of the axes system for the reaction force and, as mentioned previously, adjusted appropriately so that the forces and free moment correspond to the required laboratory system in both sense and identity. Some baseline correction may also have to be applied to compensate for any small bias in the AD converter.

Calibration

Although the force platform system is robust and relatively easy to use, it is also complex and users should always be concerned about the accuracy of their data; the accuracy of force data is established by the process of calibration. Hall *et al.*, 1996, have declared their surprise that users of force platform systems appear to give little consideration to establishing the accuracy of the tool they use. This is almost certainly due to the fact that it is not easy to do, particularly for dynamic forces, and the perception that the force platform is a robust system (for example it is not uncommon for force platforms of over 25 years old still to be in serviceable condition). The force platform system is factory calibrated before delivery but this does not include the AD converter or software processing, and the influences of installation and local environment. Some manufacturers do offer a calibration service which can be performed onsite, although this is a relatively expensive service for most laboratories to fund, particularly if they have several force platforms.

Another issue is that for at least some of the force platform variables, accuracy depends on operating conditions. For example, while the force components (Fx, Fy and Fz) are dependent only on the performance of the individual load cells (and thus the variables most likely to be accurate) the centre of pressure (Ax and Az) is dependent on the force level, force direction and force location on the platform surface. As the free moment (My) is also dependent on the centre of pressure location, this too is susceptible to operating conditions. In other words, these variables do not have a constant level of accuracy which can be established and so the effect of operating conditions on their accuracy also needs to be determined.

A favoured method for calibrating the vertical force axis *in situ* is to apply a dead weight of known value (i.e. previously calibrated). Several investigators (Bobbert and Schamhardt, 1990; Hall *et al.*, 1996; Flemming and Hall, 1997; Middleton *et al.*, 1999) have reported this approach in one way or another. Generally this is quite easy to accomplish and enables the whole measurement system to be checked. Calibration of the horizontal axes is more difficult. Hall *et al.*, 1996, proposed a pulley system whereby the calibrated force produced by a suspended dead weight is directed horizontally by a system of frictionless pulleys. They addressed the question of the real effect of cross-talk in typical gait data and reported that even with a cross-talk of one per cent (within manufacturer's specification) a large vertical force can produce a disproportionate effect on the smaller horizontal forces, such that in a typical case the cross-talk error in the horizontal data could exceed 17 per cent.

Their calibration method enabled them to evaluate the cross-talk between channels and as a result provide regression equations to reduce the effect of this on the final measured values. Using such a method they were able to establish both that their force platform was within the error tolerance specified by the manufacturers, and that that the corrected force variables were much less affected by cross-talk.

The accuracy of the centre of pressure co-ordinates (Ax and Az) has also been of some concern. Bobbert and Schamhardt, 1990, checked the accuracy of the centre of pressure co-ordinates both by applying vertical loads of up to 2000 N at various locations across the platform surface, and by using a participant to run over the platform. They reported that for static testing, a vertical load of 1000 N or more was required to ensure that the centre of pressure co-ordinates were stable, although their accuracy depended on the distance from the centre of the platform. The average error over all points was 3.5 mm (short side of the platform) and 6.3 mm (long side of the platform) although errors of up to 10 mm were found within the confines of the load cells, and up to 20 mm error if forces were applied outside the boundaries of the load cells. Similar results were obtained for the running test, suggesting that dynamic performance can be extrapolated from static testing. Bobbert and Schamhardt, 1990, proposed a numerical method to reduce the errors, although the specific solution may not be generally applicable to other types of force platform. Recently, Middleton et al., 1999, investigated the effect of separating the applied load, as would occur for example when a person was standing with both feet on the force platform. Under these conditions they reported much smaller errors. Using an AMTI force platform system Chockalingham et al., 2002, found that a threshold of 113 N was required in order to obtain a centre of pressure co-ordinate value to within a distance of 0.3 mm of its mean value. Although this represents greater accuracy than suggested by other authors, they also found that the accuracy deteriorated toward the edges of the platform.

Although a dynamic calibration is difficult to undertake, it has been attempted recently by Fairburn et al., 2000, who suggested a method based on an oscillating pendulum. The advantage of this approach is that if the inertial properties of the pendulum are known, the theoretical force can be compared to the measured force. Although the mass of the pendulum used was only 20 kg, interestingly they found no significant difference between the theoretical and measured forces for the vertical direction, but did for the horizontal direction. This may have something to do with the cross-talk problem referred to by Hall et al., 1996, that was discussed earlier.

It appears that calibration of the vertical force axis is easily conducted and should be incorporated into the measurement protocol. Calibration of the other force platform variables appears to be more complex, although the point load application method proposed by Chockalingham et al., 2002, appears to be a suitable method for easily establishing centre of pressure co-ordinate accuracy. Other more complex systems have been used, which together with regression equations seem able to improve deficiencies due to cross-talk or centre of pressure location. The accuracy of the free moment (My) does not appear to have been addressed directly, although a simple method based on a calibrated torque wrench may provide a first approach to this problem.

Applications

General force platform operation

The available software controls the operation of the force platform and the immediate data processing, although the user will have to make some choices. The main choices required relate to the range of force measurement and the sample rate. The range of force measurement needs to be appropriate for the activity and unless unduly low (for example a small child) or unduly large (for example when recording a long or triple jump) the default range is usually sufficient. It is worth looking out for telltale signs that the chosen range is incorrect, such as erratic values for centre of pressure co-ordinates Ax and Az (range too large) or a flattening in the Fy force (range too small). A second choice to be made is sample rate. Much has been said about this in the past but nowadays AD converters and computer storage capacity and processing speed are sufficiently high in performance for this to not be an issue. Sample rates of 500–2000 Hz are seen in the contemporary literature, but a sample rate of 1000 Hz represents a common choice. It should be noted however that aliasing (where the higher frequency is reflected and seen as a lower frequency in the data) may occur due to the higher frequencies that might be present in the signal. These higher frequencies are normally removed by electronic filtering before AD conversion as they cannot be removed once the data has been digitised. However, unless the force platform mounting is problematic (as noted earlier) these higher frequencies usually have very low amplitude and are therefore not a problem to the user.

Interpretation of force variables

The force platform can yield six measurement variables by equations 4.1–4.6, as described earlier. Normally these variables are presented as a time domain signals as illustrated in Figure 4.4 for a typical running stride during the support period. In this example the participant is running along the positive X axis of the force platform and uses a right foot contact. The largest of the forces is almost always the vertical support force, Fy. This force needs to be interpreted with regard to the movement, and in running we see two support peaks, the first representing the heel strike, the second representing the drive off. It should be remembered that the force value reflects the changes in motion of the centre mass of the body, but that this is not a fixed point in the body. Thus, if we were to stand on the force platform and raise or lower the arms with the rest of the body stationary, this action would affect the position of the centre of mass of the body, and hence we would expect to see a change in the vertical support force recording. The change in force does not necessarily mean that the whole body is affected, just some part of it–in this case the arms. Similarly, the impact made during heel strike is due to the lower limb decelerating rapidly, rather than the whole body (for more detail see Bobbert et al., 1992). This concept can also be nicely shown by comparing accelerations measured at the foot with those measured at the head. Some of the impact vibration is transmitted through the body but its phase and amplitude are changed.

The second largest force is the friction force in the anteroposterior (forward–backward) direction of motion. Usually, and certainly for running, movement takes place approximately along one of the platform's axes. If the force platform is located such that the person is running along the long axis X, the Fx force represents the friction force acting in the anteroposterior direction. This appears as a large negative region followed by a large positive region. This is interpreted as a negative braking force, acting from heel strike through to mid-stance, followed by a positive propulsive force from mid-stance through to toe-off. Because movement can be made in both directions (i.e. along the positive X axis as well as along the negative X axis) the horizontal force can also change its sign. Thus if the person was to run in the direction of the negative X axis, the force signal would be reversed, i.e. a large positive region, followed by a large negative region. This does not mean the force is acting differently, just that the direction of movement has changed. This is a source of confusion for some people, so care should be taken to record the direction of motion to aid interpretation later.

The third force, Fz, is the mediolateral (side-to-side) force (assuming the movement takes place as stated above) and is also a friction force, representing how the foot makes contact with the ground during the support phase. Because movement is much lower in this direction (we don't move much from side-to-side when running forward) the force is also lower, compared to Fx and Fy. It also tends to be a more rapidly changing signal and as a consequence more difficult to interpret. While the force may represent the real events taking place during contact, at least some of the force will be the result of cross-talk from the Fy channel. Assuming that the cross-talk is as specified by the manufacturer at one per cent, a vertical force of 2000 N would cause an error of 20 N in the Fz force, which is over 50 per cent for the data presented in Figure 4.4. As this will occur during the rapidly rising force levels associated with heel strike, at least some of the oscillation noted in Fz during this period is likely to be due to cross-talk. As a result, care should be taken when interpreting mediolateral forces.

In some movements, such as cutting manoeuvres, the movement is not aligned with the direction of the platform axes so it may be advisable to compute the resultant friction force as the sum of the two horizontal component forces following equation 4.7.

$$\text{Resultant Friction} = \sqrt{(Fx^2 + Fz^2)} \tag{4.7}$$

The centre of pressure co-ordinates Ax and Az are only interpretable when Fy exceeds a specified level. The artefact in these two variables can be seen in Figure 4.4d and 4.4e where the values at the start and end of contact are not well defined. Once the variable has stabilised it is possible to interpret it and for Ax we can see that this starts negative and gradually increases, as the force is applied firstly on the rear of the foot and then progresses to the front of the foot. Incidentally, the difference in value between start and finish should approximate the length of the foot, which provides a quick check for accuracy of interpretation. Similarly, the variable Az represents the movement of force

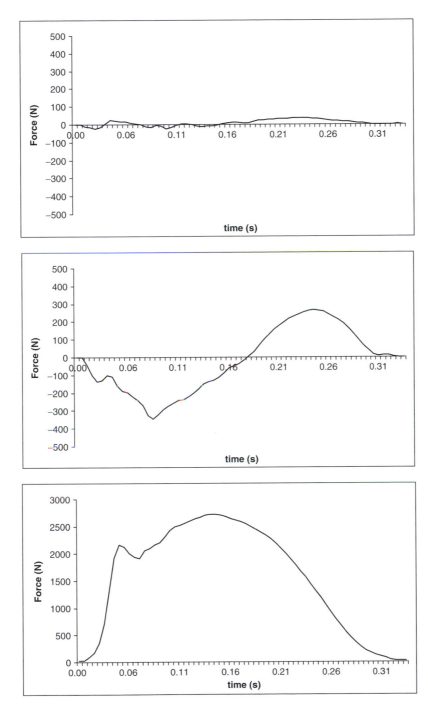

Figure 4.4   Typical force data for *Fx*, *Fy*, *Fz*, *Ax*, *Az* and *My* for a running stride

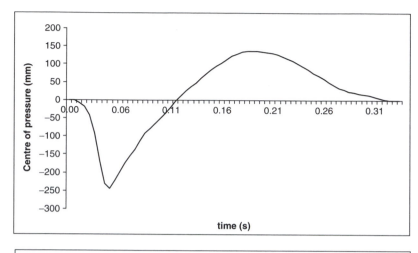

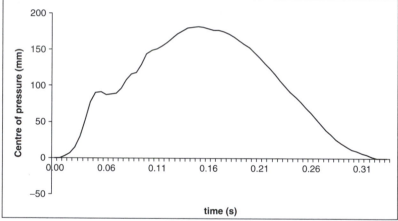

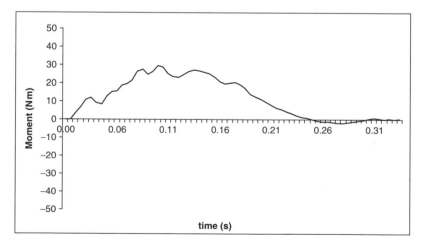

Figure 4.4   Continued

across the foot from the lateral border of the heel towards the medial border of the first metatarsal. Again, care should be taken in interpretation, as the foot is rarely placed along the force platform axis (it usually abducts, i.e. toes-out) and so the variables Ax and Az will be inter-related.

The free moment, My, represents the friction torque applied to the foot as the foot twists during contact with the ground. The fact that the foot twists during drive-off can be seen from the area of wear on well-used running shoes. For a normal runner, there will be a roundish wear area under the ball of the foot, indicating relative movement (twist) of the foot and ground during drive-off. The rapid oscillations at the start of the support phase represent the rapidly changing conditions during impact as well as the effects of cross-talk noted earlier. As My is derived from both Fx and Fz forces (see equation 4.6) this variable is likely to be affected by the problems of cross-talk. The slower change in My during drive-off can be interpreted as the external rotation twist as mentioned above. There are relatively little free moment data presented in the literature but the reader is directed to Nigg, 1986, and Holden and Cavanagh, 1991, for some useful normative data.

While detailed interpretation of the force variables can be undertaken by viewing the time history of each, interpretation can be aided by representing data in a two or three dimensional graphical format. Software packages linked to motion analysis systems can also display force data as well as motion data in a visually attractive way (Figure 4.5).

Derived force platform variables

The time history of each of the six force variables can be further quantified to provide measurement variables that might be of some use in further analysis.

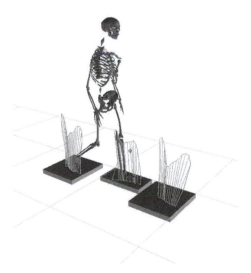

Figure 4.5 Typical graphical representation of force variables (*Fx*, *Fy*, *Fz*, *Ax* and *Az*). Note that *My* is not represented in this format

For the vertical force curve, *Fy*, variables typically of interest are the duration of contact and the magnitude of the first and second peaks. In addition, some derived force platform variables are useful such as the impulse and load rate. The impulse refers to the area under the force–time curve and can be computed by dedicated integration software or programmed using a high-level language or spreadsheet. Choice of integration routine is a relevant consideration. In the past, Simpson's rule has been useful but with the high sample rates commonly used nowadays, the trapezium rule is quite adequate. Over a number of samples *N*, the area under the force–time curve is given as

$$\text{Area} = \sum_{i=1 \text{ to } N} (F_i + F_{i+1}) \frac{\Delta t}{2} \tag{4.8}$$

Where F_i = the value for force at period *i*, and Δt = the time interval between data samples. This variable is most useful when applied to the horizontal anteroposterior force component. The negative area represents the braking impulse while the positive area represents the drive-off (propulsive) impulse. At constant running speed the two areas should be similar. If the drive-off impulse is greater than the braking impulse the runner is accelerating. Conversely, if the braking impulse is greater than the drive-off impulse, the runner is slowing down. These data can be used to check if a participant is altering their stride pattern in order to hit the force platform.

The rate of force change (or loading rate) is also of interest to the sport and exercise biomechanist, as this represents the shock imposed on the musculo-skeletal system during the impact associated with heel strike (Hennig *et al.*, 1993; Laughton *et al.*, 2003). There are various ways loading rate may be calculated, ranging from the average slope between arbitrary levels of the peak force (say 20 to 90 per cent), to the instantaneous value obtained from differentiation of the force curve. Woodward *et al.*, 1999, have recently investigated the effects of several computational methods used for the determination of loading rate. They found that the method most sensitive to differences between two clinical groups was the differentiation method based on the central difference formula (equation 4.9).

$$\text{Loading rate at point } i = (F_{i+M} - F_{i-M})/(2\,M\Delta t) \tag{4.9}$$

where *M* is the spread of data points either side of the central point (*i*). They found that the loading rate reduced as *M* increased but values of $M = 1\text{–}19$ could be used.

Computing kinematics from force data

The force recorded by the force platform represents the movement of the centre of mass. It is therefore possible to compute the acceleration, velocity and displacement of the centre of mass from force platform data. Consider a person crouched on the force platform in the process of performing a vertical jump (Figure 4.6).

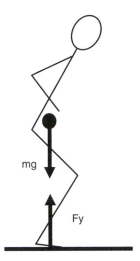

Figure 4.6   Free body diagram of a person performing a vertical jump

By using only the vertical forces acting on the centre of mass (mg) and the feet (Fy), the net force acting on the person is:

$$F_{net} = Fy - mg \tag{4.10}$$

but as $F_{net} = ma$ (from Newton's Second law)

then $a = F_{net}/m \tag{4.11}$

and as acceleration is related to the change in velocity from initial (v_i) to final (v_f)

$$v_f = v_i + at \tag{4.12}$$

and velocity is related to change in displacement from initial (d_i) to final (d_f)

$$d_f = d_i + vt \tag{4.13}$$

Equations 4.11, 4.12 and 4.13 enable us to compute the acceleration, velocity and displacement of the person, respectively, from the net force acting. Care should be taken about the process of integration used (see earlier discussion) and also the initial conditions (see Vanrenterghem *et al.*, 2001 for more detail). If a recording of a force is made during a real vertical jump the data presented in Figure 4.7 can be obtained:

There are a number of observable features in Figure 4.7 that are of interest:

- The shape of the acceleration curve is identical to that of the force curve except it is smaller by a factor of the performer's mass ($a = F/m$).
- The velocity peak of around 2.5 m s^{-1} is reached just before take-off.
- The displacement reaches a peak midway through the flight phase.
- There is some elevation of the centre of mass at take-off.

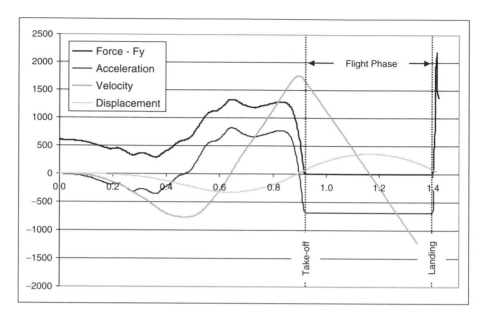

Figure 4.7 Derived acceleration, velocity and displacement data for the vertical jump. Units: force (N); acceleration (m s^{-2}) × 70; velocity (m s^{-1}) × 700; displacement (m) × 1000

- The minimum position of the centre of mass is associated with zero velocity and a high level of force (this represents an isometric contraction).
- During the flight phase the force is zero.
- The largest and most rapidly changing forces are during impact at landing.

It is quite remarkable that so much information can be obtained from a single force variable. The use of this approach is perhaps one of the most reliable methods for obtaining information on height jumped (Street *et al.*, 2001). These authors highlighted the sources of error associated with this method, although these can be reduced by taking careful precautions (see Vanrenterghem *et al.*, 2001).

Other uses of force platform data

We have seen that the force variables can be used on their own, processed to obtain derived variables, and integrated to obtain centre of mass kinematic quantities. In addition to these uses, force platform data are also widely used for computations of internal joint kinetics. This requires the collection of body joint data through the process of motion analysis. These data can be combined with the force data to compute net joint forces and moments. This is most widely seen in gait analysis and is becoming much more common as integrated motion and force analysis systems become more affordable and popular. The process by which these variables are computed is beyond the scope of this chapter, but the interested reader is referred to Nigg and Herzog, 1994; Bartlett, 1999, and Chapter 7 of this text.

PRESSURE DISTRIBUTION MEASUREMENTS

Another technique to measure kinetic aspects of human locomotion involves the use of sensors to monitor pressure distribution during ground contact, rather than the net loading profile obtained from the force platform. The force is spread over an area of contact; not concentrated at one specific point of application (i.e. centre of force). Typically, its distribution can be measured using a large array of small force sensors (e.g. each 5 mm^2) that pinpoint the areas of high pressure and provide a distribution of loading across the contact area. The summation of these distributed forces should equal the magnitude of the normal force measured by the force platform.

Although the majority of plantar pressure research has focused upon clinical problems such as the diabetic and rheumatoid foot (Lundeen *et al.*, 1994), this measurement tool has been applied in a variety of other areas including the evaluation of athletic shoe design and the influence of orthotics on foot function (Hughes, 1991; Hennig and Milani, 1995; McPoil *et al.*, 1995). Pressure systems can either be floor-mounted or in the form of a shoe insole, but there are flexible, compliant sensor arrays that can measure loading in situations involving other interfaces. These include seat pressure distribution, hand grip pressure and pressure at the residual limb–prosthesis interface of amputees during walking. Tissue areas at high risk of damage or injury can be identified because often they are continually loaded (with a high pressure-time integral) and they also tend to have excessive peak pressures with associated high loading rates. Loading can be re-distributed by interventions such as modifications in the prosthetic limb fit or its alignment. For pressure at the foot–shoe interface, athletic shoe design can be customised and any improved re-distribution of plantar pressure (with reduced high pressure 'hot spots') can be measured with an insole system under real conditions during sport and exercise activities (see Figure 4.8). The sports shoe manufacturer can control the intervention directly and modify it appropriately. Plantar pressure distribution measurements in athletes can assist in the optimisation of technique, and help to reduce the risk of foot injury. In addition, the localised loading profile allows better modelling of the forces acting on the foot and the subsequent determination of kinetic information related to performance enhancement (e.g. Stefanyshyn and Nigg, 1997).

For all applications, researchers must be aware of the expected range of the signal and select the measurement transducer and amplifier range accordingly. Manufacturers should assist in this process and offer adjustments in material properties and design of the sensors so that there is no risk of sensor overload. In addition, the construction of the sensor may only allow it to respond to a limited range of input force frequencies. This frequency response characteristic can be a limiting factor particularly if high loading rates are expected. The various types of sensors used for pressure distribution measurements have been well documented (e.g. Nigg, 2006), and the most frequently used in sport and exercise biomechanics research are the capacitance and conductance type. These are multi-layered material transducers with capacitance sensors comprising two conductive sheets separated by a thin layer of non-conducting, dielectric material; with conductance sensors having

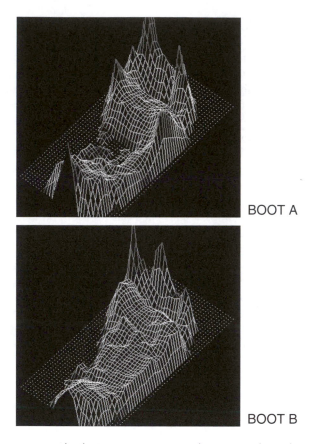

BOOT A

BOOT B

Figure 4.8 Plantar pressure distribution measurements inside two soccer boots during landing from a maximal jump in the same participant. Higher pressures under the ball of the forefoot (towards the top of each pressure contour map), where studs are located, are experienced while using boot A

a conductive polymer separator between the two conductive sheets. Both types of sensor are responsive to normal forces but horizontal shear forces are not detected. They can be manufactured into sheets or arrays of independent, equal area cells and constructed much like a circuit board. For insole devices, thin conductive strips carry signals to a small connecting box or amplifier worn above the participant's ankle. A common problem associated with the calibration of both these types of sensors is that there is not usually a straight-line relationship between sensor output response and increasing load; it is highly non-linear. Routinely, manufacturers provide users with a calibration curve as part of their software; however, this can be affected by various problems discussed later such as heat and humidity (Cavanagh *et al.*, 1992). In addition, the non-linearity often gives rise to high hysteresis qualities of the sensors, meaning that there are differences in the output signal, for any specific value of the pressure, when it is reached during increasing or decreasing pressure changes.

For a given application there may be both advantages and disadvantages of using one of the two sensor types described. In general, capacitance sensors are likely to have lower hysteresis and improved accuracy compared to conductance sensors. But they tend to be less flexible (Nigg, 2006) and sometimes, for arrays with high spatial resolution (number of sensors per unit area), sampling frequency can be limited with the commercial systems currently available. Conductance sensors may have high hysteresis and non-linear properties and, therefore, care must be taken with obtaining accurate calibration curves from the manufacturer. These sensors can offer a flexible measurement array with usually a combination of both good spatial and temporal resolution (sample rate). An example application of a conductance sensor insole system used to distinguish cushioning protection in soccer boots can be seen in Figure 4.8. Here it was necessary to have both good spatial resolution of the sensors in order to locate the pressure hot spots due to stud locations, and a high sampling rate (500 Hz) in order to adequately capture the rapid increases in pressure at the heel and forefoot regions when landing from the jump. Recently, manufacturers have tried to improve the accuracy of conductance sensor arrays by placing the sensor mat on top of a force platform (similar to the approach of Giacomozzi and Macellari, 1997). The force platform then acts as a dynamic calibrator with the pressure mat outputs adjusted to match its normal force readings. One drawback that does influence some types of conductance sensors is that sensitivity can change over time if the conductive polymer of the sensor deteriorates.

For pressure sensing systems with arrays of sensors, multiplexing tech-niques are used to reduce the need for individual cables to each sensor in the array. This can limit the sampling rate though and therefore it is important to be aware of how fast the foot loading profiles are expected to change for your intended application. For example, if the intention is to measure the in-shoe pressure distribution during sprinting, where rapid pressure peaks are expected within a foot–ground contact time of around 120 ms, then you may need a sampling rate of at least 100 Hz (approx. 12 data points) to adequately record the time of occurrence and magnitude of those pressure peaks. Sampling at 25 Hz would only provide three data points for the entire duration of contact and consequently the true loading peaks would be missed. Therefore, it becomes a challenge of matching expected signal frequency with the sampling frequency of the measurement system. As for most measurement systems, sampling frequency should be at least four times the highest frequency content of the signal. Researchers have suggested that pressure data collected between 45 and 100 Hz were adequate for walking (e.g. McPoil *et al.*, 1995) and most commercially available systems offer sampling rates between 50 and 100 Hz. For higher-speed activities, such as running, sampling frequencies of 200 Hz or greater are often required.

One method of overcoming the problem of low sample rate is to use individual or discrete pressure transducers fixed at specific anatomical locations on the plantar surface of the foot. Typically, these will include the key loading areas under the heel and ball of the foot (metatarsal heads). Discrete sensors are not multiplexed and their individual analogue signals can be sampled at high rates. However, as pressure will not be measured in some areas of the foot, the normal ground reaction force curve (as measured by a force platform) cannot be readily reconstructed. Discrete sensors can be piezoceramic, which have the added advantage of good linearity and low hysteresis, which, together with the high sample rate ability, can be an attractive pressure sensor option. Unfortunately, the piezoceramic sensors usually have significant dimensions and they can feel like small stones under the foot. Protrusion of the sensor into the plantar soft tissues causes a localised elevation in pressure (point loading artefact) due to the presence of the sensor itself (Lake *et al.*, 1991). Such distortion of the pressure distribution can be minimised by encapsulating the sensors in a layer of silicon rubber that is the same thickness as the sensor. Changes in pressure pattern caused by the measurement system are not restricted to the use of discrete sensors. Some instrumented insoles (sensor array) can behave like a layer of cushioning material that acts to smooth out and reduce the pressure peaks slightly.

Another key question is how many sensors per unit area (the spatial resolution) are required to capture the true peak pressures and/or loading area? Sensors will measure the average pressure over the whole sensor surface and therefore a force applied to a large sensor will not provide the same pressure reading as the same force applied over a small sensor. For small anatomical structures that produce a defined pressure peak (e.g. the metatarsal heads) larger sensors will underestimate the real pressure values due to the lower pressures around the peak (Lord, 1997). Considering the large variations in the size of the metatarsal heads, hallux, and toes based on foot size, the resolution of the pressure measurement system becomes an important consideration for the biomechanist. Davis *et al.*, 1997, advise that sensor sizes should be below 6.4 mm medio-laterally by 6.2 mm anterior-posteriorly in order not to underestimate actual pressures in the recording of plantar pressure patterns. Furthermore, when taking measurements on children, a higher spatial resolution of the pressure-sensing array is desirable due to the smaller size of the foot and its skeletal structures (Rosenbaum and Becker, 1997).

The use of in-shoe data collection methods is thought to eliminate the problem of targeting (where participants have abnormal foot contact on a floor-mounted pressure mat because they try to land exactly on it) because all the individual is required to do is walk normally with a pressure insole inside their shoe (Woodburn and Helliwell, 1996). Parts of the plantar pressure loading profile in an insole device can be split into specific key loading areas (e.g. metatarsal head locations) called masks in order to facilitate the numerical comparison between footwear conditions or perhaps determine the influences of training/rehabilitation. However, Shorten *et al.*, 1999, demonstrated that this analysis approach might not adequately describe any redistribution of plantar pressure because some loading data are usually discarded. Instead of applying masks, they processed data from all cells of a pressure sensitive insole on a cell-by-cell basis. Individual cell data were averaged over multiple step cycles and used for statistical comparison between experimental conditions. This was reported to provide a much-improved evaluation of pressure distribution changes.

Although they appear to offer a beneficial alternative to pressure mats, sensor insoles are more susceptible to mechanical breakdown because cables connecting the sensors to the data logger can be bent or stretched as they exit the shoe and individual sensors can also be damaged by continuous repetitive loading (Cavanagh *et al.*, 1992). Such breakage can be a result of the same areas of the insole being repeatedly subjected to high pressures. Also, the hot, humid, and usually contoured environment within the shoe can affect the reliability and validity of measurements. The effect of temperature is a key issue to be aware of when using insole systems, as it has been stated that using an in-shoe system is like placing the sensors in a 'heat chamber'. It has been found that during a 7 km run the temperature of a midsole can increase by up to 15°C (Cavanagh *et al.*, 1992). Increased temperatures affect the calibration curve of the sensors thus increasing the likelihood of inaccurate results. Finally, there can also be artifacts in the data due to bending of the insole. Bending may cause the sensors to produce an output that is unrelated to the actual foot pressure, and this problem is particular prevalent during the late part of the gait cycle when the individual pushes off the ground and the forefoot bends. In summary, when purchasing an in-shoe system, attention must be paid to the robustness of the sensor array, the fragility of the connections between sensors and the resistance to factors such as increased temperature and bending.

In conclusion, pressure distribution systems allow valuable kinetic information to be recorded for both foot–ground interaction and other loads acting on the body. Some of the key issues in selecting a pressure measurement system for a specific application have been discussed and it is clear that some care might be needed to match sensing arrays to the characteristics of the loads expected. If possible, the expected signal frequency and range should be determined before deciding for example, which sensor type and sampling frequency might be required. It is expected that with the continued development of pressure distribution measurement devices, some of the guidelines and precautions outlined here may soon become unnecessary or redundant and there will be even more widespread usage in sports and exercise biomechanics.

REPORTING A FORCE OR PRESSURE ANALYSIS STUDY

Information on the following should always be included when reporting a study involving force or pressure data analysis:

Force platform

- Manufacturer and model of the system (including dimensions of the force plate and type of amplifier).
- Manufacturer, model and resolution of the AD Converter used to sample data.
- Method of calibration (any user modification of manufacturer calibration curves).
- Sampling frequency.

Pressure sensing arrays

- Manufacturer and model of the system.
- Spatial resolution (number of sensors per cm^2).
- Sampling frequency.
- Maximum loading range (with any sensor material or design modifications).
- Size of array or number of sensors.
- Thickness of the sensors.
- Resistance to bending artifact (given as a radius of curvature).
- Description of the interface where pressure is being measured.

Processing and analysing force and pressure data

- Spatial alignment of force platform reference system to global co-ordinate system.
- Method used to synchronise the force or pressure transducers with other data acquisition systems (if used).
- Manufacturer and version of software used for processing data.
- Details of any masks used to define regions for pressure analysis.
- Method used to smooth/filter the data.
- Method used to obtain any derivative data (e.g. loading rate).
- Definitions of the dependent variables (parameters) being quantified, including their SI units.

REFERENCES

Bartlett, R.M. (1997) *Introduction to Sports Biomechanics*, London: E & FN Spon.

Bartlett, R. (1999) *Sports Biomechanics: Reducing Injury and Improving Performance*, London: E & FN Spon.

Bobbert, M.F. and Schamhardt, H.C. (1990) 'Accuracy of determining the point of force application with piezoelectric force plates', *Journal of Biomechanics*, 23: 705–710.

Bobbert, M.F., Yeadon, M.R. and Nigg, B.M. (1992) 'Mechanical analysis of the landing phase in heel-toe running', *Journal of Biomechanics*, 25: 223–234.

Cavanagh, P.R. (ed.) (1990) *Biomechanics of Distance Running*, Champaign, IL: Human Kinetics.

Cavanagh, P.R., Hewitt, F.G. and Perry, J.E. (1992) 'In-shoe plantar pressure measurement: a review', *The Foot*, 2: 185–194.

Chockalingham, N., Giakas, G. and Iossifidou, A. (2002) 'Do strain gauge platforms need in situ correction?', *Gait and Posture*, 16: 233–237.

Davis, B.L., Cothren, R.M., Quesada, P., Hanson, S.B. and Perry, J.E. (1997) 'Frequency content of normal and diabetic plantar pressure profiles: Implications foe the selection of transducer sizes', *Journal of Biomechanics*, 29: 979–983.

Fairburn, P.S., Palmer, R., Whybrow, J., Felden S. and Jones, S. (2000) 'A prototype system for testing force platform dynamic performance', *Gait and Posture*, 12: 25–33.

Flemming, H.E. and Hall, M.G. (1997) 'Quality framework for force plate testing. Journal of Engineering in Medicine', 211: 213–219.

Giacomozzi, C. and Macellari, V. (1997) 'Piezo-dynamometric platform for a more complete analysis of foot-to-floor interaction', *IEEE Transactions in Rehabilitation Engineering*, 5(4): 322–330.

Hall, M.G., Flemming, H.E., Dolan, M.J., Millbank, S.F.D. and Paul, J.P. (1996) 'Technical note on static in situ calibration of force plates', *Journal of Biomechanics*, 29: 659–665.

Hennig, E.W., Milani, T.L. and Lafortune, M. (1993) 'Use of ground reaction force parameters in predicting peak tibial accelerations in running', *Journal of Applied Biomechanics*, 9: 306–314.

Hennig, E.M. and Milani, T.L. (1995) 'In-shoe pressure distribution for running in various types of footwear', *Journal of Applied Biomechanics*, 11: 299–310.

Holden, J.P. and Cavanagh, P.R. (1991) 'The free moment of ground reaction in distance running and its changes with pronation', *Journal of Biomechanics*, 24: 887–897.

Hughes, J., Pratt, L. and Linge, K. (1991) 'Reliability of pressure measurements: the EMED F system', *Clinical Biomechanics*, 6: 14–18.

Lake, M.J., Lafortune, M.A. and Perry, S.D. (1991) 'Heel plantar pressure distortion caused by discrete sensors', in R.N. Marshall, G.A. Wood, B.C. Elliot, T.R. Ackland and P.J. McNair (eds) *Proceedings of the XIIIth Congress on Biomechanics*, pp. 370–372, Perth: International Society of Biomechanics.

Laughton, C.A., McClay-Davies, I. and Hamill, J. (2003) 'Effect of strike pattern and orthotic intervention on tibial shock during running', *Journal of Applied Biomechanics*, 19: 153–168.

Lord, M. (1997) 'Spatial resolution in plantar pressure measurement', *Medical Engineering and Physics*, 19: 140–144.

Lundeen, S., Lundquist, K., Cornwall, M.W. and McPoil, T.G. (1994) 'Plantar pressures during level walking compared with other ambulatory activities', *Foot Ankle International*, 15: 324–328.

Middleton, J., Sinclair, P. and Patton, R. (1999) 'Accuracy of centre of pressure measurement using a piezoelectric force platform', *Clinical Biomechanics*, 14: 357–360.

McPoil, T.G., Cornwall, M.W. and Yamada, W. (1995) 'A comparison of two in-shoe plantar pressure measurement systems', *Lower Extremity*, 2: 95–103.

Nigg, B.M. (1986) *The Biomechanics of Running Shoes*, Champaign, IL: Human Kinetics.

Nigg, B.M. (2006) 'Pressure distribution', in B.M. Nigg and W. Herzog (eds) *Biomechanics of the Musculo-skeletal System*, Chichester: Wiley Publishers.

Nigg, B. and Herzog, W. (1994) *Biomechanics of the Musculo-skeletal System*, Chichester: Wiley Publishers.

Rosenbaum, D. and Becker, H.P. (1997) 'Plantar pressure distribution and measurements. Technical background and clinical applications', *Foot and Ankle Surgery*, 3: 1–14.

Shorten, M., Xia, B., Eng, T. and Johnson, D. (1999) 'In-shoe pressure distribution: an alternative approach to analysis', in E. Hennig and D. Stefanyshyn (eds) *Proceedings of the IVth Footwear Biomechanics Symposium*, Canmore: International Society of Biomechanics.

Stefanyshyn, D.J. and Nigg, B.N. (1997) 'Mechanical energy contribution of the metatarsophalangeal joint to running and sprinting', *Journal of Biomechanics*, 30 (11): 1081–1085.

Street, G., McMillan, S., Board, W., Rasmussen, M. and Heneghan, J.M. (2001) 'Sources of error in determining countermovement jump height with impulse method', *Journal of Applied Biomechanics*, 17: 43–54.

Vanrenterghem, J., De Clercq, D. and Van Cleven, P. (2001) 'Necessary precautions in measuring correct vertical jumping height by means of force plate measurements', *Ergonomics*, 44: 814–818.

Woodward, C.M., James, M.K. and Messier, S.P. (1999) 'Computational methods used in determination of loading rate: experimental and clinical implications', *Journal of Applied Biomechanics*, 15: 404–417.

Woodburn, J. and Helliwell, P.S. (1996) 'Observations on the F-Scan in-shoe pressure measuring system', *Clinical Biomechanics*, 11: 301–305.

CHAPTER 5

SURFACE ELECTROMYOGRAPHY

Adrian Burden

INTRODUCTION

Electromyography is a technique used for recording changes in the electrical potential of muscle fibres that are associated with their contraction. The fundamental unit of the neuromuscular system is the motor unit, which consists of the cell body and dendrites of a motor neuron, the multiple branches of its axon, and the muscle fibres that it innervates. The number of muscle fibres belonging to a motor unit, known as the innervation ratio, ranges from about 1:6 (e.g. extraocular muscles) to 1:1900 (Enoka, 2002). Detailed descriptions of the generation of an action potential by a motor neuron, its propagation along a muscle fibre and the processes that convert it into force within the fibre are beyond the scope of these guidelines and are more than adequately covered elsewhere (e.g. Enoka, 2002, and Luttman, 1996). Knowledge of these processes is, however, paramount as the biomechanist needs to understand the nature of the detected signal. In addition, and in agreement with Clarys and Cabri, 1993, a detailed knowledge of musculo-skeletal anatomy is also essential to ensure that electrodes are placed over the correct muscles.

The signal that is detected using surface electrodes is complex and is best understood by considering its underlying waveforms. The following terms originate from those introduced by Winter *et al.*, 1980, and describe such waveforms as they develop from single action potentials into the detected signal. A muscle fibre action potential or a motor action potential (MAP) is the waveform detected from the depolarisation wave as it propagates in both directions along a muscle fibre. The waveform detected from the spatio-temporal summation of individual MAPs originating from muscle fibres belonging to a motor unit in the vicinity of a pair of recording electrodes is termed a motor unit action potential (MUAP). A motor unit action potential train (MUAPT) is the name given to the waveform detected from the repetitive sequence of MUAPs (i.e. repeated motor unit firing). Finally, the total signal seen at the electrodes is called the myoelectric signal (Winter *et al.*, 1980), electromyographic signal (Basmajian and De Luca, 1985) or interference pattern (Enoka, 2002). This is the algebraic summation of all MUAPTs within the detection volume of the electrodes, and is represented schematically in Figure 5.1. The electromyographical signal when amplified and recorded, is termed the electromyogram (EMG).

Whilst these terms are useful in understanding the complex nature of the raw EMG, it is obvious that a single MAP could not be recorded using even the smallest surface electrodes. Individual MUAPs can, however, be identified from EMGs recorded using indwelling electrodes by a process known as decomposition (a review of the methods and applications of EMG decomposition can be found in De Luca and Adam, 1999 and Stashuk, 2001). More recently, promising steps have been made in identifying individual MUAPs from EMGs recorded using a linear array of tiny surface electrodes (e.g. Merletti *et al.*, 2001; 2003). Unlike the electrodes used in linear arrays, those that are used in the recording of EMGs from relatively large, superficial muscles during sport and exercise are typically greater than 1 cm in diameter (circular electrodes) or length (rectangular electrodes). In addition, the muscle fibres of different motor units tend to overlap spatially (Cram and Kasman, 1998), which means that a given region of muscle could contain fibres from between 20 and 50 different motor units (Enoka, 2002). Thus, normal surface electrodes have the potential to detect MUAPTs from many different motor units, as depicted in Figure 5.1.

The above explanation presents the oversimplified view that only the number of active motor units and their firing rates can affect the EMG. In reality, a host of other anatomical, physiological and technical factors also have the potential to influence the electromyographical signal (e.g. Basmajian and De Luca, 1985; De Luca and Knaflitz, 1990; De Luca, 1997 and Cram and Kasman, 1998). Most recently, De Luca, 1997, provided a comprehensive review of such factors and grouped them as causative, intermediate and deterministic.

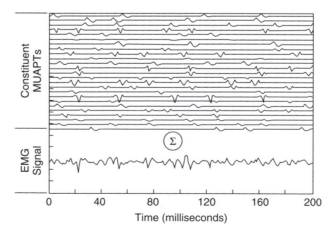

Figure 5.1 An EMG signal formed by adding (superimposing) 25 mathematically generated motor unit action potential trains (from Basmajian and De Luca, 1985)

The causative factors have a fundamental influence on the EMG and were further divided by De Luca, 1997, into extrinsic and intrinsic groups. Extrinsic factors include, for example, the area and shape of the electrodes, the distance between them, and their location and orientation. Intrinsic factors include, for example, fibre type composition, muscle fibre diameter, their depth and location with regard to the electrodes, and the amount of tissue between the surface of the electrodes and the muscle; in addition to the number of active motor units. The intermediate factors, which are influenced by one or more of the causative factors, include the detection volume of the electrodes, their filtering effect, and cross-talk from neighbouring muscles. Finally, the deterministic factors, which are influenced by the intermediate factors and have a direct influence on the recorded EMG, include the amplitude, duration and shape of the MUAPs. The biomechanist has little influence over the intrinsic (causative) factors that can affect the EMG. However, the extrinsic (causative) factors are affected both by the techniques used by the biomechanist and their choice of equipment.

Basmajian and De Luca, 1985, Cram and Kasman, 1998 and Clarys, 2000, have all previously documented the birth of electromyography in the eighteenth century and its development into the twentieth century. In general, electromyography has developed in two directions. Clinical electromyography is largely a diagnostic tool used to study the movement problems of patients with neuromuscular or orthopaedic impairment, whereas kinesiological electromyography is concerned with the study of muscular function and co-ordination during selected movements and postures (Clarys and Cabri, 1993 and Clarys 2000). Since the 1960s (e.g. Broer and Houtz, 1967) a plethora of sport-and exercise-related studies have been published (Clarys and Cabri, 1993 and Clarys, 2000). The majority of such studies have investigated when muscles are active and the role that they play in complex sports and exercises, and how muscle activity is altered by training and skill acquisition. Surface electromyography is also now used to predict individual muscle force-time histories (e.g. Hof, 1984; Dowling, 1997 and Herzog et al., 1999) and to quantify muscular fatigue (e.g. De Luca, 1997).

A number of other books, chapters and review articles relating to kinesiological electromyography have been published since the mid-1970s. Some of the more recent texts (e.g. De Luca and Knaflitz, 1990; Winter, 1990; Soderberg and Knutson, 1995; Kumar and Mital, 1996; De Luca, 1997; Cram and Kasman, 1998; Gleeson, 2001 and Clancy et al., 2002) have, like Basmajian and De Luca, 1985, before them, provided a generic discussion of methods, applications and recent developments in surface electromyography. The majority of these sources have provided extensive coverage of the methods used to record and process EMGs. The following sections compare commercially available surface electromyography systems as well as methods that are currently used by researchers and practitioners. Particular attention is paid to aspects of methodology that have not received sufficient attention previously, such as the reduction of cross-talk and the normalisation of processed EMGs. Recommendations are made based on information from the texts listed above, other scientific literature, and both the International Society of Electrophysiology and Kinesiology (ISEK) (Winter et al., 1980 and

Merletti, 1999) and the SENIAM Project (Hermens *et al.*, 1999); as well as the author's own experiences.

EQUIPMENT CONSIDERATIONS

It is generally accepted that the peak amplitude of the raw EMG recorded using surface electromyography does not exceed 5 mV and that its frequency spectrum is between 0–1000 Hz (e.g. Winter, 1990); with most of the usable energy limited to below 500 Hz and the dominant energy between 50–150 Hz (De Luca, 2002). When detecting and recording EMGs a major concern should be that the fidelity of the signal is maximised (De Luca, 1997). This is partly achieved by maximising the signal-to-noise ratio (i.e. the ratio of the energy in the electromyographical signal to that in the noise). Noise can be considered as any signals that are not part of the electromyographical signal and can include movement artifacts, detection of the electrocardiogram, ambient noise from other machinery, and inherent noise in the recording equipment. Details of these, and other, sources of noise are beyond the scope of these guidelines and are adequately covered elsewhere (e.g. Örtengren, 1996; Cram and Kasman, 1998). In particular, Clancy *et al.*, 2002, provides very useful recommendations for reducing noise from a variety of sources. Maximising the fidelity of the EMG is also achieved by minimising the distortion (i.e. alteration of the frequency components of the signal) that it receives during detection, amplification and recording (De Luca, 2002). Both the equipment and procedures used to detect and record EMGs have a major influence on their fidelity, and should be given careful consideration.

Most commercially available electromyographical systems can be classified as either hard-wired, telemetry or data logger systems, with some companies offering more than one of these options. A data logger or telemetry system is necessary if data are to be collected away from the main recording apparatus; however data loggers typically do not allow on-line viewing of EMGs as they are being recorded and telemetry systems can be prone to ambient noise and can not be used in areas with radiated electrical activity. Hardwired systems don't suffer from these limitations, but obviously preclude data collection outside of the vicinity of the recording apparatus. Table 5.1 details companies that manufacture electromyography systems including the characteristics of the amplifiers that they use. The fidelity of the recorded electromyogram is dependent on these characteristics and, as such, should be a major consideration when purchasing a system. Whilst a detailed explanation of amplifier characteristics is beyond the scope of these guidelines (for details see Basmajian and De Luca, 1985; Winter, 1990; Cram and Kasman, 1998 and Clancy *et al.*, 2002) the important ones are listed below, together with recommended requirements; which are generally agreed upon by De Luca, 1997, and the SENIAM Project (Merletti *et al.*, 1999a):

- Input Impedance (>100 MΩ)
- Common Mode Rejection Ratio (CMRR) (>80 dB [10 000])

Table 5.1 Summary of amplifier characteristics for commercially available electromyography systems

Company	System	Amplifier					
	Name	Type	Gain*	Bandwidth (Hz)	CMRR† (dB)	Input impedance (MΩ)	Input referred noise (μV)‡
B & L Engineering	MA–300	Hard-wired	P 330	12–>5000	95	>100	
Biometrics	SX230 (DataLog)	Data logger	P 1K M 0.3–1K	20–450	>96	10 000 000	<5
	SX230 (DataLink)	Hard-wired	P 1K M 0.3–1K	20–450	>96	10 000 000	<5
Biopac	EMG100C	Hard-wired	M 500 1K, 2K, 5K	1, 10, 100 –500, 5000	110	1000	0.2 rms
	TSD150		P 350	12–500	95	100	
Bortec	AMT	Hard-wired	P 500, 2K M 100–15K	10–1000	115	10000	4.5 rms
DelSys	Bagnoli	Hard-wired	P 10 M 100, 1, 10K	20–450	>92	100 000 000	1.2 rms
Glonner	MyoMonitor	Data logger	P 1K	20–450	>92	100 000 000	1.5 rms
	BioTel	Telemetry		Up to 2000			
MIE	MT8	Telemetry	P 1K, 4K, 8.6K M 1–5	12–1000	>110	>10	<4
Mega	Data Logger	Data logger	P 1K, 4K, 8K	6–6000	>110	>10	<4
	ME6000	Data logger & Telemetry		8–500, 15–500	110		
	NeurOne	Hard-wired		0–200	>110		
	NeurOne Matrix WBA	Data logger Telemetry		100–10000	>120		0.5 rms

Continued

Table 5.1 Cont'd

Company	System Name	Type	Amplifier Gain*	Bandwidth (Hz)	CMRR† (dB)	Input impedance (MΩ)	Input referred noise (μV)‡
Motion Lab Systems	MA–300	Hard-wired	P 20 or 300 M 200–10K	20–2000	>100	100	<1.2 rms
Noraxon	MYOTRACE 400	Hard-wired & Telemetry		20–500			
	TELEMYO2400T	Telemetry		10–500	>100	>100	<1 rms
	TELEMYO2400TG2	Telemetry			>100	>100	<1 rms
	MYOSYSTEM1200	Hard-wired		10–500	>100	>100	<1 rms
	MYOSYSTEM1400	Hard-wired		10–500	>100	>100	<1 rms
Run Technologies	MQ-8	Telemetry		2–450	>90	1000	1
	Myopac	Hard-wired	M 1K, 2K, 5K, 10K	10–1000	90	1	<0.8 rms
	Myopac Jr.	Hard-wired	M 1K, 2K, 5K, 10K	10–1000	90	1	<0.8 rms
Zebris Medical GmbH	EMG 4	Hard-wired	M 1, 2.5, 5K	7.5–1000	110	1 000 000	0.28 p-p
	EMG 8	Hard-wired	M 1, 2.5, 5K	7.5–1000	110	1 000 000	0.28 p-p
	EMG 8 Bluetooth	Telemetry		7–500	110	1 000 000	0.28 p-p

Notes
*P = preamplifier, M = main amplifier
†CMRR = common mode rejection ratio
‡rms = root mean square, p-p = peak-to-peak

- Input Referred Noise ($<$1–2 μV rms)
- Bandwidth (20–500 Hz)
- Gain (variable between 100 and 10 000; see Sampling)

Whilst the requirements of amplifiers are generally agreed on by biomechanists, the configuration of electrodes and the material from which they are made are not. The SENIAM Project (Freriks *et al.*, 1999) prefers pre-gelled Ag/AgCl electrodes that are circular with a diameter of 10 mm and a centre-to-centre distance of 20 mm; such as that used by Bortec (see Table 5.2). In contrast, De Luca, 1997, recommends silver bar electrodes that are 10 mm long, 1 mm wide, have a distance of 10 mm between them and are attached without the use of a gel; such as that used by Delsys. Despite these and a host of other types of electrodes being commercially available (see Table 5.2), only De Luca, 1997, appears to provide a rationale for his recommendation. If the inter-electrode distance is increased the bandwidth of the detected electromyographical signal will decrease, and vice versa. Assuming that the conduction velocity of the depolarisation wave along a muscle fibre is 4 m s^{-1}, an inter-electrode distance of at least 1 cm will result in a bandwidth that contains the full frequency spectrum of the raw EMG (for further explanation see Basmajian and De Luca, 1985).

DATA COLLECTION PROCEDURES

Electrode configuration, location and orientation

Contrary to earlier recommendations it is now universally agreed that, in order to maximise the amplitude of the detected signal, the electrodes should not be placed either side of and at the same distance from a motor point, which usually coincides with the innervation zone. Differential amplifiers subtract the signal detected by one electrode from that detected by the other. Thus, locating electrodes either side of a motor point will lead to the cancellation of symmetrical action potentials that are travelling in opposite directions from the neuromuscular junction and that reach the electrodes at approximately the same time (e.g. Merletti *et al.*, 2001). This is illustrated in Figure 5.2 by using the concept of single MAP detected by a pair of electrodes from a linear array (electrode pair and EMG number 2). However, if both electrodes are placed to one side of a motor point the signal is not cancelled to the same extent, as one electrode detects the MAP slightly earlier than the other (e.g. electrode pair and EMG number 3 in Figure 5.2).

Based on the above, it is generally agreed that electrodes should be located between a motor point and a tendon (e.g. De Luca, 1997 and Freriks *et al.*, 1999). Figure 5.2 also illustrates the use of an array of electrodes, rather than a single pair, to locate motor points (Merletti *et al.*, 2001; 2003). In the absence of a linear electrode array or a stimulator to detect the location of motor points, electrodes can be placed in the centre of the belly of the muscle whilst under contraction (Clarys and Cabri, 1993).

Table 5.2 Summary of sensor characteristics for commercially available electromyography systems

Company	Name	Channels	Material	Shape	Size	Inter-electrode	Type
B & L Engineering	MA-300	6, 10, 16	Steel	Disk	$1/2''$	$13/16''$ & $1\ 3/8''$	Re-usable
Biometrics	SX230 (DataLog)	8	Steel	Disk	10 mm	20 mm	Re-usable
	SX230 (DataLink)	8	Steel	Disk	10 mm	20 mm	Re-usable
Biopac	EMG100C						Re-usable
	TSD150		Ag/AgCl	Disk	11.4 mm	20 or 35 mm	Pre-gelled
Bortec	AMT	8, 16	Ag/AgCl	Disk	10 mm	20 mm	Re-usable
DelSys	Bagnoli	4, 8, 16	Ag	Bar	10 × 1 mm	10 mm	Re-usable
	MyoMonitor	8, 16	Ag	Bar	10 × 1 mm	10 mm	Re-usable
Glonner	BioTel	1–4, 8–32					
MIE	MT8	8	Ag/AgCl	Rectangle	30 × 20 mm	Variable	Pre-gelled
	Data Logger	8	Ag/AgCl	Rectangle	30 × 20 mm	Variable	Pre-gelled
Mega	ME6000	4, 16					
	NeurOne	4					
	NeurOne Matrix	2					
	WBA						
Motion Lab Systems	MA-300	6, 10, 16	Steel	Disk	12 mm	18 mm	Re-usable
Noraxon	MYOTRACE 400	2	Ag/Ag/Cl	Disk	10 mm	20 mm	Pre-gelled
	TELEMYO2400T	4, 8	Ag/Ag/Cl	Disk	10 mm	20 mm	Pre-gelled
	TELEMYO2400TG2	4, 8, 12, 16	Ag/Ag/Cl	Disk	10 mm	20 mm	Pre-gelled
	MYOSYSTEM1200	1–8	Ag/Ag/Cl	Disk	10 mm	20 mm	Pre-gelled
	MYOSYSTEM1400	1–16	Ag/Ag/Cl	Disk	10 mm	20 mm	Pre-gelled
Run Technologies	MQ-8	2					
	Myopac	16					
	Myopac Jr	8					
Zebris Medical GmbH	EMG 4	4					
	EMG 8	4					
	EMG 8 Bluetooth	8					

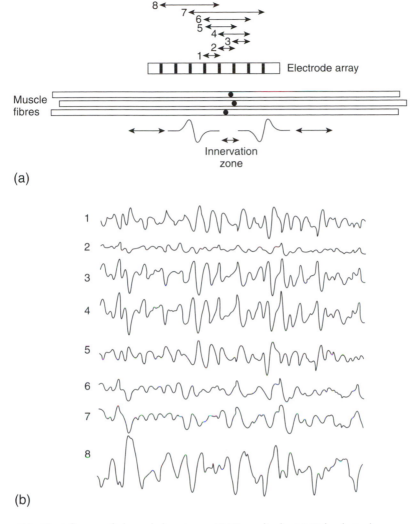

Figure 5.2 The influence of electrode location on EMG amplitude. (a) Eight electrodes arranged in an array, with a 10 mm spacing between each electrode. The lines (numbered 1 to 8) above the array indicate the different combinations of electrodes that were used to make bi-polar recordings. Inter-electrode distances are 10 mm for pairs 1, 2 and 3; 20 mm for pairs 4 and 5; 30 mm for pair 6; 40 mm for pair 8; and 50 mm for pair 7. (b) EMGs recorded using the array shown in (a) when placed on the skin overlying the biceps brachii at 70 per cent of MVC (adapted by Enoka, 2002 from Merletti *et al.*, 2001)

However, it should be recognised that this location could coincide with that of a motor point.

Recommended guidelines for locating electrode placement sites over specific muscles also continue to be published (e.g. Zipp, 1982; Cram *et al.*, 1998; Freriks *et al.*, 1999). Virtually all major, superficial muscles are now covered by such guidelines, which typically locate electrodes about a point that is a specific distance along a line measured between two anatomical landmarks.

Clarys and Cabri, 1993, warned against using such recommendations for anything other than isometric contractions. If they are used, it should not be as a substitute for a good knowledge of musculo-skeletal anatomy and the correct location should always be confirmed using voluntary activation of the muscle of interest and palpation. Following the location of an appropriate site, it is universally agreed that, if possible, the electrodes should be oriented along a line that is parallel to the direction of the underlying muscle fibres (e.g. De Luca, 1997 and Freriks et al., 1999).

Skin preparation

The high input impedance that is offered by many of today's amplifiers (see Table 5.1) has diminished the need to reduce the skin–electrode impedance to below levels around $10 \, k\Omega$. Skin preparation techniques that involve abrasion with fine sandpaper or scratching with a sterile lancet (e.g. Okamoto et al., 1987) are, therefore, now largely redundant. Some preparation of the skin (to below $55 \, k\Omega$) is, however, still necessary in order to obtain a better electrode–skin contact and to improve the fidelity of the recorded signal (e.g. Cram and Kasman, 1998; Freriks et al., 1999 and Hewson et al., 2003). Typically, this involves cleaning the skin with soap and water and dry shaving it with a disposable razor. Additional rubbing with an alcohol-soaked pad and then allowing the alcohol to vapourise can be used to further reduce impedance, although this should be avoided when using participants with fair or sensitive skin. Cram and Kasman, 1998, and Freriks et al., 1999, report further details of modern skin preparation techniques.

In addition to the recording electrodes, differential amplifiers require the use of a reference, or ground, electrode that must be attached to electrically neutral tissue (e.g. a bony landmark). The degree of skin preparation given to the reference electrode site should be the same as that afforded to the muscle site. Some commercially available systems (e.g. Delsys) use a single, remote reference electrode for all muscle sites whilst others (e.g. MIE) use more local sites for each separate muscle that is being investigated. These latter systems usually have each pre-amplifier mounted on the press stud on the reference electrode and have relatively short leads between the pre-amplifier and the detecting electrodes. This sometimes precludes the reference electrode from being located over, for example, a bony landmark; particularly when investigating long muscles of the upper and lower extremities (e.g. hamstrings).

Most biomechanists also advise using an electrode gel or paste to facilitate detection of the underlying electromyographical signal (e.g. Cram and Kasman, 1998). This can be accomplished either through the use of pre-gelled electrodes (Freriks et al., 1999) or by applying a gel or paste to the skin or electrode prior to attachment (Clancy et al., 2002). Use of gel or paste is not always necessary when using so called 'active electrodes' i.e. those that are mounted onto the pre-amplifier. Here, the electrolytic medium is provided by the small amount of sweating that takes place when dry electrodes are applied to the skin (Cram and Kasman, 1998 and Clancy et al., 2002).

Cross-talk

Even if surface electrodes are placed close to the belly of the muscle it is possible that the detected signal may contain energy that emanates from other, more distant muscles. This form of noise, known as cross-talk, has been reported to be as high as 17 per cent of the signal from maximally activated nearby muscles, in both the lower (De Luca and Merletti, 1988) and upper leg (Koh and Grabiner, 1992). Despite more recent research suggesting that cross-talk may not be as serious a problem as previously thought (e.g. Solomonow *et al.*, 1994 and Mogk and Keir, 2003), it is still an issue that biomechanists should address and attempt to reduce as much as possible. This is particularly pertinent when recording EMGs from muscles that are covered by thicker than normal amounts of subcutaneous fat, such as the gluteals and abdominals (Solomonow *et al.*, 1994).

The presence of cross-talk has traditionally been detected using functional tests (e.g. Winter *et al.*, 1994) or cross-correlation techniques (e.g. Winter *et al.*, 1994 and Mogk and Keir, 2003). Functional tests (also known as manual muscle tests) involve getting the participant to contract muscles that are adjacent to the one under investigation, without activating the one of interest. The detection of a signal from electrodes overlying the muscle of interest is, therefore, an indication of cross-talk. Whilst this technique has been found to provide an indication of the presence of cross-talk by the author, it is susceptible to two main limitations of which the biomechanist should be aware. The participant may not be able to activate nearby muscles, as pointed out by De Luca, 1997; or the muscle of interest may be (moderately) activated in the process of trying to contract adjacent ones. Cross-correlation is a statistical technique that essentially quantifies the magnitude of any common component that is present in two separate signals i.e. from the muscle of interest and an adjacent one suspected of contributing to cross-talk; with a higher correlation indicating a stronger presence of cross-talk. Despite being criticised by De Luca, 1997, it is still used by researchers to detect cross-talk (e.g. Mogk and Keir, 2003). Two further techniques for detecting the presence of cross-talk have been proposed by De Luca, 1997. One involves comparing the frequency spectrum (see Processing EMGs in the Frequency Domain) of an EMG signal that is suspected of containing cross-talk with that of one believed to be primarily from the muscle of interest. The signal from a muscle further away from the electrodes would experience greater spatial (low pass) filtering than that from a muscle located directly below the electrodes. Thus, an EMG signal suspected of containing cross-talk would be expected to have a frequency spectrum that is more compressed towards the lower frequencies. The other technique involves using surface electrodes on muscles that are adjacent to the one of interest and wire electrodes in deep muscles, to monitor them for (lack of) activity. This approach is cumbersome and uses wire-electrodes, which may not be available.

Decreasing the size of the electrodes or the spacing between them reduces the chances of recording cross-talk (e.g. Koh and Grabiner, 1993 and Winter *et al.*, 1994). However, the use of excessively small inter-electrode distances will alter the bandwidth of the signal and may, therefore, compromise its fidelity. In addition, altering the size and spacing of the electrodes is often not possible due to the standard configuration used by some manufacturers (e.g. Bortec and Delsys). Research has shown that the most effective way of reducing cross-talk to almost negligible levels is to use the 'double differential technique' (De Luca and Merletti, 1988 and Koh and Grabiner, 1993). Prior to this section, the discussion of equipment considerations and data collection procedures has referred to the use of a single pair of electrodes per muscle site (in addition to the reference electrode). In the vast majority of commercially available recording systems the electrodes are attached to a single differential amplifier (often referred to simply as a differential amplifier) that calculates the difference between the signals detected by each electrode overlying the muscle of interest. The amplifier used in the double differential technique has three, rather than two, detecting electrodes that are equally spaced apart, which calculates the difference between the signals detected by electrodes one and two, and electrodes two and three. These two new (single differentiated) signals are then further differentiated (double differentiation) by the amplifier (for further details refer to De Luca, 1997). This procedure works by significantly decreasing the detection volume of the three electrodes, and thereby filtering out signals from further away (De Luca, 1997). To the author's knowledge the double differential technique only exists in two commercially available systems (Delsys and Motion Lab Systems). It is envisaged that other manufacturers will follow suit in the future and the double differential amplifier will be an option in all major recording systems.

Sampling

The Nyquist Theorem dictates that electromyographical signals which are detected using surface electrodes should be sampled at a minimum of 1000 Hz (ideally 2000 Hz) to avoid aliasing (i.e. loss of information from the signal). Sampling of the signal into a PC should also use an analogue-to-digital-converter (ADC) that has at least 12 bits (ideally 16 bits) to ensure that as small a change in muscle activity as possible is able to be detected by the system. Prior to recording EMGs caution should be exercised over selection of the gain of the pre-amplifier/amplifier. Of primary concern is that too high a gain is not chosen, which may result in the amplified signal exceeding the output voltage of the system (typically ±5 V). This is evidenced by 'clipping' (i.e. a raw signal that has had its negative and positive peaks chopped off at a specific amplitude), which often occurs when a very high gain (e.g. 10,000) is used for a muscle that typically emits a large signal (e.g. tibialis anterior). Care must also be taken not to use too low a gain (e.g. 100), as this may result in only a small part of the output voltage being utilised and hence small changes in signal amplitude not being quantified; particularly if a low resolution ADC is used (i.e. 12 bits or less). Ideally, a gain should be selected that utilises as much of the output voltage of the system as possible, whilst avoiding clipping. This typically ranges between 1,000 and 5,000 for superficial muscles in sport and exercise applications when using an output voltage of ±5 V. Most systems include pre-amplifiers with different gains (e.g. MIE) or a choice of gain settings on the main amplifier (e.g. Delsys) to enable selection of an appropriate value.

The reader is referred to Merletti *et al.*, 1999a; Clancy *et al.*, 2002 and De Luca, 2003, for a more in depth discussion of the issues surrounding sampling of electromyographical signals.

PROCESSING, ANALYSING AND PRESENTING ELECTROMYOGRAMS

Processing EMGs in the time domain

Raw EMGs have been processed in numerous ways, particularly since the advent of computers (see Basmajian and De Luca, 1985 and Winter, 1990). Today, raw EMGs are processed in the time domain almost exclusively using either the Average Rectified EMG, Root Mean Square or Linear Envelope. All of which provide an estimate of the amplitude of the raw EMG in μV or mV.

The Average Rectified EMG (AREMG, e.g. Winter *et al.*, 1994) has also been termed the Average Rectified Value (ARV, e.g. Merletti *et al.*, 1999a), Mean Absolute Value (MAV, e.g. Clancy *et al.*, 2002), and the Mean Amplitude Value (MAV, e.g. Merletti *et al.*, 1999a); but will be referred to as the ARV in this chapter. Calculation of the ARV involves first either removing all of the negative phases of the raw EMG (half-wave rectification) or reversing them (full wave rectification). The latter option is preferred, and almost exclusively performed today, because it retains all of the energy of the signal (Basmajian and De Luca, 1985). The integral of the rectified EMG is then calculated over a specific time period, or window (T), and the resulting integrated EMG is finally divided by T to form the ARV (see equation 5.1). The integrated EMG (reported in μVs or mVs) was a common processing method in its own right from the latter half of the twentieth century (see Winter, 1990). However, despite the ARV being similar to and providing no additional information to the integrated EMG the latter method is mainly used to provide an estimate of the total amount of activity.

$$\text{ARV} = \frac{1}{T} \int_0^T |X(t)| \, dt \tag{5.1}$$

where: $X(t)$ is the EMG signal.

T is the time over which the ARV is calculated.

The Root Mean Square EMG (RMS) is the square root of the average power of the raw EMG calculated over a specific time period, or window (T) (see equation 5.2).

$$\text{RMS} = \sqrt{\frac{1}{T} \int_0^T X^2(t) dt} \tag{5.2}$$

Both the ARV and RMS are recognised as appropriate processing methods by De Luca's group (e.g. Basmajian and De Luca, 1985 and De Luca and Knaflitz, 1990), the SENIAM Project (Merletti *et al.*, 1999a), as well as other authors (e.g. Clancy *et al.*, 2002). The same authors also prefer the RMS over the ARV, albeit for different reasons. De Luca (1997) states that the ARV is a measure of the area under the rectified EMG and thus has no specific physical meaning. In comparison, the RMS is a measure of the power of the signal and thereby has a clear physical meaning. Merletti *et al.*, 1999a, claim that for a stationary signal, which may occur during a low level isometric contraction, the RMS shows less variability than the ARV when calculated over successive time windows. Thus, the RMS has the potential to detect signal changes that could be masked by the greater variability of the ARV.

Rather than using a single calculation of the RMS or ARV, the raw EMG is often processed by making successive calculations throughout its duration. The resulting series of values form a type of moving average (for further details see Winter *et al.*, 1980 or Basmajian and De Luca, 1985). Regardless of which method is used, the biomechanist also needs to decide on the duration (or width) of the successive time windows (T). Basmajian and De Luca, 1985, recommend choosing a width between 100 and 200 ms. Merletti *et al.*, 1999a, further recommend that for a sustained isometric contraction, durations of 0.25–2 s are acceptable, with shorter widths (0.25–0.5 s) used for contraction levels above 50 per cent MVC and longer ones used (1–2 s) for lower level contractions. The smaller the width of the time window the less smooth the resulting curve will be (Basmajian and De Luca, 1985). Thus, for constant level isometric contractions a width of short duration will result in relatively high variability between values calculated over successive windows. Use of a larger window width would result in a smoother curve, for which the variability of successive values will be lower (Merletti *et al.*, 1999a).

The moving average approach (using either RMS or ARV) described above is also used to analyse raw EMGs recorded from dynamic contractions, where the aim is often to detect (sometimes rapid) changes in muscle activity. Selection of short duration window widths (e.g. 10–50 ms) may allow the detection of rapid alterations in activity, but the resulting curve will still resemble the rectified EMG. Thus, peak amplitudes from repetitions of the same task will remain highly variable. Adoption of longer widths (e.g. 100–200 ms) will reduce the variability of peak amplitudes, but the resulting curve will lose the trend of the underlying EMG. As such, rapid changes in muscle activity may go undetected. A possible solution is to use a moving average (either RMS or ARV) in which the time windows overlap instead of including discrete sections of the EMG (for further details see Winter *et al.*, 1980 or Basmajian and De Luca, 1985). Overlapping the windows by a progressively greater amount results in a curve that increasingly follows the trend of the underlying rectified EMG, but without the variable peaks that are evident in the rectified EMG.

The Linear Envelope is also still a popular processing method, and is recommended by Merletti *et al.*, 1999a, for use on EMGs from dynamic contractions. Similar to the moving average, this involves smoothing the rectified EMG with a low pass filter (for further details see Winter *et al.*, 1980 or Winter 1990), and also results in a curve that follows the trend of the EMG.

When using the Linear Envelope, the type, order and cut-off frequency of the filter need to be decided on. Traditionally, a second order Butterworth filter has been applied (e.g. Winter *et al.*, 1980) with a cut-off frequency that has ranged between 3 and 80 Hz (Gabel and Brand, 1994). Deciding on the cut-off frequency is similar to choosing the width and amount of overlap of the time window when using a moving average. Use of a low cut-off frequency will result in a very smooth curve, which will be unable to detect rapid changes in activation. Conversely, choice of a higher frequency will closely follow rapid changes in activity, but will still bear the peaks that characterise the rectified EMG. For further details of amplitude processing methods and their effect on the electromyographical signal the reader should refer to Clancy *et al.*, 2002.

Threshold analysis

Following processing the EMG is often used to estimate when a muscle is active (i.e. on) or inactive (i.e. off). Typically, in order to determine the amplitude threshold at which the muscle is considered to be active, the baseline EMG (or noise) is treated as a stochastic variable. The mean of this baseline is, for example, calculated over 50 ms and the muscle is deemed to be active when the EMG amplitude exceeds three standard deviations above the mean baseline activity for 25 ms or more (Di Fabio, 1987). Numerous variations of these parameters have been proposed, and recently reviewed by Hodges and Bui, 1996; Allison, 2003 and Morey-Klapsing *et al.*, 2004. In agreement with Di Fabio, 1987, Hodges and Bui, 1996, discovered that a sample width of 25 ms more accurately identified the onset of muscle activity, in relation to a visually determined value, than either 10 ms or 50 ms. They also reported that use of three standard deviations above mean baseline activity increased the risk of failing to identify EMG onset when it occurred (i.e. a Type II error), and delayed onset determination in relation to using two standard deviations. Following on from the discussion in the previous section, the degree of smoothing to which the EMG is subjected to during (time domain) processing will also affect the correct identification of EMG onset (Hodges and Bui, 1996 and Allison, 2003). Use of a Linear Envelope with a cut-off frequency of 50 Hz was discovered by Hodges and Bui, 1996, to result in a more accurate determination of muscle activity onset than either 10 Hz or 500 Hz.

A more conservative threshold of two standard deviations. above the mean has also been included in recent recommendations (e.g. De Luca, 1997). Furthermore, for the muscle of interest to be considered to be either on or off the amplitude should exceed or fall below the threshold for a period that is greater than the physiological conditions that limit the resolution of this on/off time (i.e. the time taken for the signal to reach the electrodes from the innervation zone) (Gleeson, 2001 and Allison , 2003). For most applications this should be at least twice this physiologically limited resolution, or 20 ms (De Luca, 1997). However, it must also be appreciated that the success of the chosen parameters in accurately and reliably detecting the onset of muscle activity will be affected by both the signal-to-noise ratio of the EMG (i.e. clean vs. noisy baseline) and the rate of increase in its amplitude during the specific task (i.e. slow vs. fast movements) (for further details see Allison, 2003). Thus, most authors (e.g. Di Fabio, 1987; Hodges and Bui, 1996 and Allison, 2003) agree that whatever the chosen method it should be supplemented by repeated visual verification.

Ensemble averaging EMGs

It is often desirable to present and analyse the average (mean) EMG patterns from a number of trials, particularly for cyclic events such as walking, running and cycling. Such a pattern of processed EMGs is termed an ensemble average (e.g. Winter *et al.*, 1980). The first stage in producing an ensemble average is to decide on a start and an end point for each trial (e.g. heel contact to heel contact of the same foot for a walking stride). The duration of each trial is then converted to a new standardised time-base (e.g. the percentage of the stride time). The process is often referred to as 'temporal normalisation' and should not be confused with amplitude normalisation, which is described in the next section. Next, data from each trial are interpolated at the same points on the new time-base, for example, 2 or 5 per cent intervals). This can be done using linear interpolation or by fitting a cubic spline to the data points. Finally, data from all trials is averaged at each of the points on the new time-base. The resulting ensemble average is typically displayed along with an appropriate measure of the variability between trials (e.g. ±1 standard deviation).

Ensemble averages can be produced for the same individual over a number of strides (i.e. intra-individual) as described above, and also for a number of individuals. An inter-individual ensemble average is created similarly by calculating the mean of the intra-individual ensemble averages at each of the points on the time-base.

Assessment of intra-individual and inter-individual variability of EMG patterns has traditionally been accomplished using either the coefficient of variation or the variance ratio (VR in equation 5.3). The coefficient of variation was promoted by Winter and colleagues throughout the 1980s and 1990s (e.g. Yang and Winter, 1984), whilst the variance ratio has sporadically been used to measure the variability of EMG patterns (e.g. Burden *et al.*, 2003) after initially being devised by Hershler and Milner, 1978. Unlike the variance ratio, the coefficient of variation is essentially the ratio of the standard deviation of the EMG patterns to the mean pattern. Therefore, the magnitude of the mean has the potential to either elevate or reduce the value of the coefficient. As a consequence, the coefficient of variation is sensitive to both the amount of smoothing applied to the EMG during processing and the number of cycles included in the ensemble average (Gabel and Brand, 1994). For these reasons the coefficient variation should not be used to compare the variability of EMG patterns from different muscles; and certainly not to compare the variability of EMG patterns with those of other biomechanical parameters. It is recommended that the variance ratio is used to assess the variability of EMG patterns, particularly when comparisons of variability are to be made across muscles, individuals etc.

$$\text{VR} = \frac{\displaystyle\sum_{i=1}^{k}\sum_{j=1}^{n}(X_{ij} - \overline{X}_i)^2 / k(n-1)}{\displaystyle\sum_{i=1}^{k}\sum_{j=1}^{n}(X_{ij} - \overline{X})^2 / (kn-1)} \tag{5.3}$$

where: k is the number of time intervals within the cycle.

n is the number of cycles (for intra-individual variability) or participants (for inter-individual variability).

X_{ij} is the EMG value at the ith time for the jth cycle or participant.

$\overline{X}_i$ is the mean of the EMG values at the ith time over the jth cycle or participant.

$\overline{X}$ is the mean of the EMG values, i.e. $\overline{X} = \dfrac{1}{k}\displaystyle\sum_{i=1}^{k}\overline{X}_i$.

Normalising EMGs

Processed EMGs can only be compared with those recorded from the same muscle without the removal of electrodes (i.e. during the same testing session). Relocation of electrodes over the same muscle on subsequent occasions will invariably result in the detection of different motor units. The skin-electrode impedance will also differ between sessions, regardless of how well skin preparation techniques are adhered to, which will affect the shape of the underlying MUAPs. These and other factors that were previously outlined in the Introduction Section will, therefore, affect the amplitude of the processed EMG. As such, the amplitude of EMGs recorded from the same muscle on different occasions, as well as from different muscles and different individuals cannot be compared directly, even if they have been processed using the same method. This problem may be solved by (amplitude) normalisation of EMGs after they have been processed. Traditionally, this has involved expressing each data point of the processed EMG from the specific task as a proportion or a percentage of the peak EMG from an isometric maximal voluntary contraction (MVC) of the same muscle that has been processed in the same way (referred to as the Isometric MVC Method). In addition to allowing the comparison of EMGs from different muscles, this normalisation method has the potential to reveal how active a muscle is during a specific task; by expressing it as a proportion or percentage of its maximal activation capacity. However, despite being recommended by both ISEK (Merletti, 1999) and the SENIAM project (Merletti et al., 1999b) the Isometric MVC Method has received several criticisms that biomechanists should be conscious of before using it.

Among others, Clarys, 2000, recognised that use of the Isometric MVC Method is limited by the poor reliability of EMGs that are recorded from MVCs. This would cast doubt on the value of comparing EMGs normalised using the Isometric MVC Method and question the capability of this method to reveal the proportion of an individual's muscle activation capacity required to perform a specific task. Because of this, the reportedly improved reliability of EMGs from sub-maximal contractions has resulted in these EMGs being used as the denominator in the normalisation equation (e.g. Yang and Winter, 1984). In particular, De Luca, 1997, advocates the use of EMGs from contractions that are less than 80 per cent MVC in order to provide a more stable reference value (referred to as the Reference Contraction Method). This method should also be used when normalising EMGs from individuals who are unable or unwilling to perform MVCs due to musculo-skeletal pain or injury. For example, Healey et al., 2005, obtained a reference contraction of the lumbar erector spinae in individuals with chronic low back pain by holding a 4 kg bar at arm's length for 15 s. A second criticism of the Isometric MVC Method centres on whether the maximal activation capacity of the muscle is actually elicited during an MVC. Outputs from this normalisation method in excess of unity (i.e. 100 per cent) indicate that the activity of the muscle during a specific task can be greater than that recorded during the isometric MVC. For example, Jobe et al., 1984, reported that EMGs from the serratus anterior were 226 per cent of the EMG from a maximal muscle test during the acceleration phase of the overarm throw. In response to this criticism, extensive research using the twitch interpolation technique has revealed that (most) individuals are able to maximally activate their muscles during isometric MVCs (e.g. Allen et al., 1995). In partial agreement with the earlier criticism of the Isometric MVC Method, the same authors do warn that the ability to consistently achieve maximal activation varied between individuals. Finally, as most tasks in sport and exercise involve non-isometric contractions a further criticism aimed at the Isometric MVC Method is whether it is appropriate to use the EMG from an isometric contraction (MVC) to normalise EMGs from dynamic contractions (tasks). Some previous studies (e.g. Mirka, 1991) reported that EMG amplitude from MVCs was affected by muscle length or the rate at which it shortened or lengthened. This would necessitate dividing each data point of the task EMG with that from a dynamic MVC that had been performed with the same muscle kinematics (referred to as the Isokinetic MVC Method, as such MVCs are usually performed on an isokinetic dynamometer). However, use of the Isokinetic MVC Method has recently been shelved by Burden and Bartlett, 1999 and Burden et al., 2003, who found only minor differences in the output of it and the Isometric MVC Method.

Based on the above information, it is recommended that if an investigation requires that EMGs be compared between sessions, muscles or individuals then they should be normalised using the Reference Contraction Method (that is ideally less than 80 per cent MVC). If the investigation is further interested in how active the muscle is (in relation to its maximal activation capacity) then the Isometric MVC Method can be used to provide an indication of this, as well as to compare EMGs. It is strongly recommended that individuals receive extensive practice in performing isometric MVCs before EMGs from them are used in the Isometric MVC Method. Previously unrehearsed MVCs will result in torque or force, and hence muscle activity, that is far from maximal.

Amplitude normalisation can also be used to reduce inter-individual variability of EMGs recorded from the same task. It is now well established that dividing each data point within the task EMG by either the mean or the peak EMG from the same task EMG (referred to as the Mean Dynamic Method and the Peak Dynamic Method respectively) is the most effective way of improving group homogeneity (e.g. Yang and Winter, 1984 and Burden *et al.*, 2003). However, due to the nature of the denominator used in their normalisation equation, the Mean and Peak dynamic methods cannot be used to compare the amplitude of EMGs from different muscles and individuals.

Processing EMGs in the frequency domain

Raw EMGs are processed in the frequency domain primarily to investigate changes in the signal that accompany muscular fatigue. It is now well established that fatigue is associated with a compression of the frequency spectrum towards the lower frequencies (see Figure 5.3), that occurs largely due to a decrease in the conduction velocity of action potentials and a consequent increase in the duration of MUAPs. The reader is referred to Basmajian and De Luca, 1985 or De Luca, 1997, for a more detailed explanation of these processes and the physiological mechanisms behind them.

Transformation of a raw EMG from the time domain to the frequency domain is typically achieved using a Fast Fourier Transform (FFT). Details of how the FFT decomposes the signal into its various frequency contributions are beyond the scope of these guidelines, and the reader is referred to Enoka, 2002 or Giakas, 2004, for further details. The FFT requires specification of the time window (or epoch) over which the spectrum is calculated and the shape of the window (e.g. rectangular or more complex such as Hanning). Merletti *et al.*, 1999a, recommend a time window of between 0.5 and 1 s, but also reveal that the window shape has little effect on parameters used to represent the frequency spectrum (see below).

The output of the FFT is typically represented as the power spectrum density (PSD), which shows the relative magnitudes of the range of frequencies present in the raw signal (see bottom of Figure 5.3). One of two parameters is commonly obtained from the PSD in order to quantify it. The median frequency (MDF) is defined as the frequency that divides the PSD into equal halves, and the mean frequency (MNF) is calculated as the sum of the product of the individual frequencies and their own power divided by the total power (e.g. Finsterer, 2001). Whilst the MNF is less variable than the MDF, the latter is less sensitive to noise and more sensitive to spectral compression (e.g. De Luca and Knaflitz, 1990; Merletti *et al.*, 1999a). As such, both SENIAM (Merletti *et al.*, 1999a) and De Luca (e.g. De Luca, 1997) recommend use of the MDF as an indicator of muscular fatigue.

Regardless of the chosen parameter, it is typically obtained from consecutive time windows, to enable changes in the signal that occur as a consequence of fatigue to be monitored. Successive values from the contraction period are

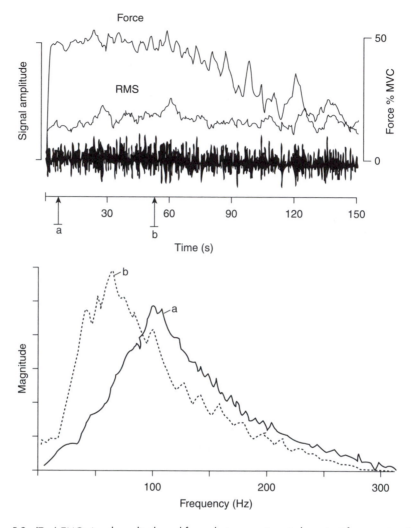

Figure 5.3 (Top) EMG signal amplitude and force during an attempted constant-force contraction of the first dorsal interosseus muscle. (Bottom) Power spectrum density of the EMG signal at the beginning (a) and at the end (b) of the constant force segment of the contraction (from Basmajian and De Luca, 1985)

then analysed using (linear) regression; with the intercept of the regression line being the initial frequency and the gradient representing the fatigue rate (e.g. Ng *et al.*, 1996). In addition to fatigue, the frequency spectrum of the raw EMG is affected by a host of other factors (see Introduction section). Similar to analysis in the time domain (see Normalising EMGs section) specific frequencies (e.g. MDF) cannot, therefore, be compared directly when they are calculated from EMGs recorded from different muscles or individuals, or from the same muscle when the electrodes have been re-applied. However, comparisons can be made between the gradient of the regression line in order to investigate differences in fatigue rates between different muscles, occasions or individuals (e.g. Ng *et al.*, 1996). Nevertheless, care should still be taken to use the same electrode configuration, location and orientation, and skin preparation and cross-talk reduction procedures whenever possible (see Data Collection Procedures).

SENIAM (Merletti *et al.*, 1999a) and De Luca (e.g. De Luca, 1997) also acknowledge that the FFT should only be used on EMGs that display high stability; typically those recorded from sustained force isometric contractions between 20 and 80 per cent MVC. EMGs recorded from dynamic contractions typically reduce the stability of the signals largely as a consequence of recruitment and de-recruitment of different motor units. As such, the FFT should only be used in such circumstances when signal stability is reasonably high and parameters (i.e. MDF or MNF) should only be calculated at the same phase of repetitive cyclic events (De Luca, 1997). The problem of obtaining spectral parameters from non-stationary signals has largely been overcome by using the joint time-frequency domain approach which estimates the change in frequency as a function of time (see Giakas, 2004 for a review). The simplest method that conforms to this approach is the short-time Fourier transform, which splits the EMG into small continuous or overlapping time windows, applies a FFT to each and calculates the MDF or MNF as above (e.g. Englehart *et al.*, 1999). Recently, more sophisticated methods of time-frequency domain analysis have been applied to EMGs. These include the Wigner-Ville transform from which the instantaneous MDF or MNF is calculated (e.g. Knaflitz and Bonato, 1999), the Hilbert transform from which the averaged instantaneous frequency is obtained (Georgakis *et al.*, 2003), and wavelet analysis which produces intensity spectra (e.g. Wakeling *et al.*, 2001). Readers are referred to Englehart *et al.*, 1999; Georgakis *et al.*, 2003 and Hostens *et al.*, 2004, for a comparison of the methods and performance of various time-frequency domain approaches.

REPORTING AN ELECTROMYOGRAPHICAL STUDY

Largely as a result of the different, and often erroneous, units and terminology used by researchers at the time, ISEK published standards (Winter *et al.*, 1980) by which electromyographical investigations should be reported. These recommendations have largely been superseded by a further standardisation document (Merletti, 1999), which is endorsed by both ISEK and the *Journal of Electromyography and Kinesiology*. The SENIAM project also published guidelines for reporting EMGs recorded using surface electromyography (Merletti *et al.*, 1999b) which are almost identical to those produced by ISEK. The following information is based largely on that provided by ISEK and the SENIAM project, and should be considered as the minimum detail required:

Equipment

- Type of system (e.g. hard-wired, telemetry)
- Manufacturer(s) and model of the system, or different components (e.g. electrodes and amplifier) of the system

- Material, size and shape of electrodes
- Type of amplifier (i.e. differential or double differential) and the following characteristics:
  - Common Mode Rejection Ratio (CMRR) (dB)
  - Input impedance (MΩ)
  - Gain
  - Input referred noise (either peak-to-peak or rms) (μV) or signal-to-noise ratio (dB)
  - Bandwidth (Hz), including details of the filter types (e.g. Chebyshev, Butterworth) and slopes of the cut-offs at each end of the bandwidth (dB/octave or dB/decade)
- Manufacturer, model and number of bits of the ADC used to sample data into the computer.

Data collection procedures

- Location of the electrodes (ideally) with respect to the motor point
- Orientation of the electrodes with respect to the underlying muscle fibres
- Inter-electrode distance
- Skin-preparation techniques, including details of any gel or paste used
- Procedures used to check for the presence of cross-talk and/or reduce the amount of cross-talk
- Sampling frequency (Hz).

Processing and analysing EMGs

- Amplitude processing
  - Method used to process the raw EMG (e.g. RMS, ARV, Linear Envelope):
    - For ARV and RMS: width of time window and (if applicable) overlap of time window
    - For Linear Envelope: type and order of filter, and cut-off frequency
  - Method used to normalise processed EMGs (e.g. Mean Dynamic, Isometric MVC, Reference Contraction), if applicable. If the Isometric MVC or Reference Contraction method was used then details of how the participants were trained to perform these contractions, their position, stabilisation methods and joint angles of involved limbs should be included
  - Threshold detection method (e.g. level and duration), if applicable
  - Details of ensemble averaging, if applicable
- Frequency processing
  - Algorithm used (e.g. FFT)
  - Length and type of window used (e.g. rectangular, Hanning)
  - Choice of parameter (e.g. MDF, MNF).

REFERENCES

Allen, G.M., Gandevia, S.C. and McKenzie, D.K. (1995) 'Reliability of measurements of muscle strength and voluntary activation using twitch interpolation', *Muscle and Nerve*, 18: 593–600.

Allison, G.T. (2003) 'Trunk muscle onset detection technique for EMG signals with ECG artefact', *Journal of Electromyography and Kinesiology*, 13: 209–216.

Basmajian, J.V. and De Luca, C.J. (1985) *Muscles Alive: Their Functions Revealed by Electromyography*, 5th edn, Baltimore: Williams & Wilkins.

Broer, R. and Houtz, J. (1967) *Patterns of Muscle Activity in Selected Sports Skills: An Electromyographic Study*, Springfield, Il.: Charles C. Thomas.

Burden, A.M. and Bartlett, R.M. (1999) 'Normalisation of EMG amplitude: an evaluation and comparison of old and new methods', *Medical Engineering & Physics*, 21: 247–257.

Burden, A.M., Trew, M. and Baltzopoulos, V. (2003) 'Normalisation of gait EMGs: a re-examination', *Journal of Electromyography and Kinesiology*, 13: 519–532.

Clancy, E.A., Morin, E.L. and Merletti, R. (2002) 'Sampling, noise-reduction and amplitude estimation issues in surface electromyography', *Journal of Electromyography and Kinesiology*, 12: 1–16.

Clarys, J.P. (2000) 'Electromyography in sports and occupational settings: an update of its limits and possibilities', *Ergonomics*, 43: 1750–1762.

Clarys, J.P. and Cabri, J. (1993) 'Electromyography and the study of sports movements: a review', *Journal of Sports Sciences*, 11: 379–448.

Cram, J.R. and Kasman, G.S. (1998) *Introduction to Surface Electromyography*, Gaithersberg, Maryland, MD: ASPEN.

Cram, J.R., Kasman, G.S. and Holtz, J. (1998) 'Atlas for electrode placement', in J.R. Cram and G.S. Kasman (eds), *Introduction to Surface Electromyography*, Gaithersberg, Maryland, MD: ASPEN.

De Luca, C. (1997) 'The use of surface electromyography in biomechanics', *Journal of Applied Biomechanics*, 13: 135–163.

De Luca, C. (2002) Surface electromyography: detection and recording. [WWW]. <http://www.delsys.com/Attachments_pdf/WP_SEMGintro.pdf> (accessed 27 August 2007).

De Luca, C.J. and Merletti, R. (1988) 'Surface myoelectric signal cross-talk among muscles of the leg', *Electroencephalography and Clinical Neurophysiology*, 69: 568–575.

De Luca, C.J. and Knaflitz, M. (1990) *Surface Electromyography: What's New?* Boston, MA: Neuromuscular Research Centre.

De Luca, C.J. and Adam, A. (1999) 'Decomposition and analysis of intramuscular electromyographical signals' in U. Windhorst and H. Johannson (eds), *Modern Techniques in Neuroscience Research*, Heidelberg: Springer.

De Luca, G. (2003) Fundamental concepts in EMG signal acquisition (Revision 2.1). [WWW]. <http://www.delsys.com/Attachments_pdf/WP_Sampling1-4.pdf> (accessed 27 August 2007).

Di Fabio, R.P. (1987) 'Reliability of computerized surface electromyography for determining the onset of muscle activity', *Physical Therapy*, 67: 43–48.

Dowling, J.J. (1997) 'The use of electromyography for noninvasive prediction of muscle forces, current issues', *Sports Medicine*, 24: 82–96.

Englehart, K., Hudgins, B., Parker, P.A. and M. Stevenson (1999) 'Classification of the myoelectric signal using time-frequency based representations', *Medical Engineering and Physics*, Special Issue: Intelligent Data Analysis in Electromyography and Electroneurography, 21: 431–438.

Enoka, R.M. (2002) *Neuromechanics of Human Movement*, 3rd edn, Champaign, IL: Human Kinetics.

Finsterer, J. (2001) 'EMG-interference pattern analysis', *Journal of Electromyography and Kinesiology*, 11: 231–246.

Freriks, B., Hermans, H.J., Disselhorst-King, C. and Rau, G. (1999) 'The recommendations for sensors and sensor placement procedures for surface elctromyography', in H.J. Hermens, B. Freriks, R. Merletti, D. Stegeman, J. Blok, G. Rau, C. Disselhorst-Klug and G. Hägg (eds), *European Recommendations for Surface Electromyography: Results of the SENIAM Project*, Enschede: Roessingh Research and Development.

Gabel, R.H. and Brand, R.A. (1994) 'The effects of signal conditioning on the statistical analyses of gait EMG', *Electroencephalography and Clinical Neurophysiology*, 93: 188–201.

Georgakis, A., Sterioulas, L.K. and Giakas, G. (2003) 'Fatigue analysis of the surface EMG signal in isometric constant force contractions using the averaged instantaneous frequency', *IEEE Transactions on Biomedical Engineering*, 50: 262–265.

Giakas, G. (2004) 'Power spectrum analysis and filtering', in N. Stergiou (ed.), *Innovative Analyses of Human Movement*, Champaign, IL: Human Kinetics.

Gleeson, N.P. (2001) 'Assessment of neuromuscular performance using electromyography', in R.G. Eston and T. Reilly (eds), *Kinanthropometry and Exercise Physiology Laboratory Manual: Tests, Procedures and Data. Volume 2: Exercise Physiology*, 2nd edn, London: Routledge.

Healey, E.L., Fowler, N.E., Burden, A.M. and McEwan, I.M. (2005) 'The influence of different unloading positions upon stature recovery and paraspinal muscle activity', *Clinical Biomechanics*, 20: 365-371.

Hermens, H.J., Freriks, B., Merletti, R., Stegeman, D., Blok, J., Rau, G., Disselhorst-Klug, C. and Hägg, G. (eds.) (1999). *European Recommendations for Surface Electromyography: Results of the SENIAM Project*. Enschede: Roessingh Research and Development.

Hershler, C. and Milner, M. (1978) 'An optimality criterion for processing electromyographic (EMG) signals relating to human locomotion', *IEEE Transactions on Biomedical Engineering*, 25: 413–420.

Herzog, W., Guimares, A.C.S and Zhang, Y.T. (1999) 'EMG', in M. Nigg and W. Herzog (eds), *Biomechanics of the Musculo-skeletal System*, 2nd edn, Chichester: Wiley.

Hewson, D.J., Hogrel, J.-Y., Langeron, Y. and Ducêne, J. (2003) 'Evolution in impedance at the electrode–skin interface of two types of surface EMG electrodes during long-term recordings', *Journal of Electromyography and Kinesiology*, 13: 273–279.

Hodges, P.W. and Bui, B.H. (1996) 'A comparison of computer-based methods for the determination of onset of muscle contraction using electromyography', *Electroencephalography and Clinical Neurophysiology*, 101: 511–519.

Hof, A.L. (1984) 'EMG and muscle force: an introduction', *Human Movement Science*, 3: 119–153.

Hostens, I., Seghers, J., Spaepen, A. and Ramon, H. (2004) 'Validation of the wavelet spectral estimation technique in biceps brachii and brachioradialis fatigue assessment during prolonged low-level static and dynamic contractions', *Journal of Electromyography and Kinesiology*, 14: 205–215.

Jobe, F.W., Radovich, D., Tibone, J.E. and Perry, J. (1984) 'An EMG analysis of the shoulder in pitching: a second report', *The American Journal of Sports Medicine*, 12: 218–220.

Knaflitz, M. and Bonato, P. (1999) 'Time-frequency methods applied to muscle fatigue assessment during dynamic contractions', *Journal of Electromyography and Kinesiology*, 9: 337–350.

Koh, T.J. and Grabiner, M.D. (1992) 'Cross-talk in surface electromyograms of human hamstring muscles', *Journal of Orthopaedic Research*, 10: 701–709.

Koh, T.J. and Grabiner, M.D. (1993) 'Evaluation of methods to minimize cross-talk in surface electromyography', *Journal of Biomechanics*, 26: 151–157.

Kumar, S. and Mital, A. (eds) (1996) *Electromyography in Ergonomics*, London: Taylor & Francis.

Luttman, A. (1996) 'Physiological basis and concepts of electromyography', in S. Kumar and A. Mital (eds), *Electromyography in Ergonomics*, London: Taylor & Francis.

Merletti, R. (1999) 'Standards for reporting EMG data', *Journal of Electromyography and Kinesiology* (all volumes).

Merletti, R., Farina, D., Hermens, H., Frericks, B. and Harlaar, J. (1999a) 'European recommendations for signal processing methods for surface electromyography', in H.J. Hermens, B. Freriks, R. Merletti, D. Stegeman, J. Blok, G. Rau, C. Disselhorst-Klug and G. Hägg (eds), *European Recommendations for Surface Electromyography: Results of the SENIAM Project*, Enschede: Roessingh Research and Development.

Merletti, R., Wallinga, W., Hermens, H.J. and Freriks, B. (1999b) 'Guidelines for reporting SEMG data', in H.J. Hermens, B. Freriks, R. Merletti, D. Stegeman, J. Blok, G. Rau, C. Disselhorst-Klug and G. Hägg (eds), *European Recommendations for Surface Electromyography: Results of the SENIAM Project*, Enschede: Roessingh Research and Development.

Merletti, R., Rainoldi, A. and Farina, D. (2001) 'Surface electromyography for noninvasive characterization of muscle', *Exercise and Sport Sciences Reviews*, 29: 20–25.

Merletti, R., Farina, D. and Gazzoni, M. (2003) 'The linear electrode array: a useful tool with many applications', *Journal of Electromyography and Kinesiology*, 13: 37–47.

Mirka, G.A. (1991) 'The quantification of EMG normalization error' *Ergonomics*, 34: 343–352.

Mogk, J.P.M. and Keir, P.J. (2003) 'Crosstalk in surface electromyography of the proximal forearm muscles during gripping tasks', *Journal of Electromyography and Kinesiology*, 13: 63–71.

Morey-Klapsing, G., Arampatzis, A. and Brüggemann, G.P. (2004) 'Choosing EMG parameters: comparison of different onset determination algorithms and EMG integrals in a joint stability study', *Clinical Biomechanics*, 19: 196–201.

Ng, J.K.-F., Richardson, C.A., Kippers, V., Parnianpour, M. and Bui, B.H. (1996) 'Clinical applications of power spectral analysis of electromyographic investigations in muscle tension', *Manual Therapy*, 2: 99–103.

Okamoto, T., Tsutsumi, H., Goto, Y. and Andrew, P. (1987) 'A simple procedure to attenuate artefacts in surface electrode recordings by painlessly lowering skin impedance', *Electromyography and Clinical Neurophysiology*, 27: 173–6.

Örtengren, R. (1996) 'Noise and artefacts' in S. Kumar and A. Mital (eds), *Electromyography in Ergonomics*, London: Taylor & Francis.

Soderberg, G.L. and Knutson, L.M. (1995) 'EMG Methodology', in R.L. Craik and C.A. Oatis (eds), *Gait Analysis: Theory and Application*, St. Louis: Mosby.

Solomonow, M., Baratta, R., Bernardi, M., Zhou, B., Lu, Y., Zhu, M. and Acierno, S. (1994) 'Surface and wire EMG crosstalk in neighbouring muscles', *Journal of Electromyography and Kinesiology*, 4: 131–142.

Stashuk, D. (2001) 'EMG signal decomposition: how can it be accomplished and used?', *Journal of Electromyography and Kinesiology*, 11: 151–173.

Wakeling, J.M., Pascual, S.A., Nigg, B.M. and von Tscharner, V. (2001) 'Surface EMG shows distinct populations of muscle activity when measured during sustained submaximal exercise', *European Journal of Applied Physiology*, 86: 40–47.

Winter, D.A. (1990) *Biomechanics and Motor Control of Human Movement*, 2nd edn, New York: Wiley.

Winter, D.A., Rau, G., Kadefors, R., Broman, H. and De Luca, C.J. (1980) *Units, Terms and Standards in the Reporting of EMG Research*, USA: International Society of Electrophysiological Kinesiology.

Winter, D.A., Fuglevand, A.J. and Archer, S.E. (1994) 'Crosstalk in surface electromyography: theoretical and practical estimates', *Journal of Electromyography and Kinesiology*, 4: 5–26.

Yang, J.F. and Winter, D.A. (1984) 'Electromyographic amplitude normalization methods: improving their sensitivity as diagnostic tools in gait analysis', *Archives of Physical Medicine and Rehabilitation*, 65: 517–521.

Zipp, P. (1982) 'Recommendations for the standardization of lead positions in surface electromyography', *European Journal of Applied Physiology and Occupational Physiology*, 50: 41–54.

CHAPTER 6

ISOKINETIC DYNAMOMETRY

Vasilios Baltzopoulos

INTRODUCTION

Isokinetic dynamometry is the assessment of dynamic muscle strength, and function in general, by measuring the joint moment exerted during constant joint angular velocity movements. It has widespread applications in sport, exercise and pathological conditions for the measurement of muscle strength, for assessment of training or rehabilitation programmes, prediction of performance, prevention of injuries and in basic research on the mechanics of muscles, tendons and joints, modelling and simulation, and many other related areas (Baltzopoulos and Brodie, 1989; Kellis and Baltzopoulos, 1995). Isokinetic dynamometers are extremely useful and unique devices that allow the assessment of dynamic muscle and joint function under specific conditions. However, there are many factors, related mainly to the biomechanical and physiological complexities of the musculo-skeletal system, that could affect the measurements. It is, therefore, important to understand the mechanical basis of the measurements and the basic biomechanics of joint motion to be able to use an isokinetic dynamometer properly.

Human movement is produced by the rotation of segments around the instantaneous axis of rotation of the joints. Mechanically, rotation is only possible with the application of a moment. Muscles generate muscle forces that are transmitted to the bones via tendons. As an example, we will consider a knee extension motion in the sagittal plane only, around an instantaneous axis of rotation that is perpendicular to the plane of the segment motion. Assuming that there is only one active muscle-tendon unit, the moment producing the rotation can be determined simply as the product of the muscle force and its shortest distance from the axis of rotation or moment arm (Figure 6.1).

In general, the angular acceleration of a rotating segment will depend on the net moment applied, according to the fundamental equation of planar

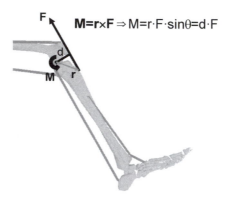

$$M = r \times F \Rightarrow M = r \cdot F \cdot \sin\theta = d \cdot F$$

Figure 6.1 The application of a muscle force *F* (N) around the axis of rotation (transmitted via the patellar tendon in this example) with a position vector *r* relative to the origin. This generates a muscle moment *M* (N m) that is equal to the cross product (shown by the symbol ×) of the two vectors (*r* and *F*). The shortest distance between the force line of action and the axis of rotation is the moment arm *d* (m). *θ* is the angle between *r* and *F*. *M* is also a vector that is perpendicular to the plane formed by *F* and *r* (coming out of the paper) and so it is depicted by a circular arrow

(two dimensional) motion for rotation:

$$\sum_{i=1}^{n} M_i = I \cdot \alpha \qquad (6.1)$$

where:

$M_1 + M_2 + \cdots + M_n$: the total or net joint moment,

I: the moment of inertia (parameter describing the distribution of the segment mass around the axis of rotation).

α: the angular acceleration of the rotating segment around the joint axis of rotation.

Muscle strength is normally defined as the maximum joint moment that can be exerted under different muscle length, velocity and action (concentric, isometric, eccentric) conditions. For this reason, the measurement of net joint moment at different joint positions, angular velocities and action conditions is essential for the assessment of muscle strength and the dynamic capabilities of the neuromuscular system in general. The maximum joint moment under such dynamic conditions is normally measured using different isokinetic dynamometer systems, so it is important to understand the operating principles of these machines and the measurement techniques used.

APPLICATIONS OF ISOKINETIC DYNAMOMETRY

Muscle and joint function assessment are essential in sport and exercise, not only for performance purposes but also for the assessment and rehabilitation of injury (Baltzopoulos and Brodie, 1989; Kellis and Baltzopoulos, 1995). Isokinetic dynamometry is one of the safest forms of exercise and testing. Once the pre-set angular velocity is attained, the resistive moment is equal to the net moment applied, so that the joint and muscles are loaded to their maximum capacity over the range of constant (isokinetic) movement. Because the dynamometer resistive moment does not normally exceed the net applied moment, no joint or muscle overloading and, therefore, risk of injury occurs.

Measurement of the joint moment, exerted at different angular velocities and joint positions, enables the establishment of moment velocity and moment position relationships for various joints in subjects from different populations. This information is essential for computer modelling and simulation of human movement (e.g. King and Yeadon, 2002) as well as for research into the physiology and mechanics of muscle (see Kellis and Baltzopoulos, 1996). Major review papers and books that describe Isokinetic Dynamometry applications in dynamic muscle strength assessment, rehabilitation and clinical problems include: Osternig, 1986; Baltzopoulos and Brodie, 1989; Cabri, 1991; Perrin, 1993; Kannus, 1994; Kellis and Baltzopoulos, 1995; Chan *et al.*, 1996; Gleeson and Mercer, 1996; Brown, 2000; De Ste Croix *et al.*, 2003; Dvir, 2004.

This chapter will discuss mainly the biomechanical aspects of isokinetic movements and measurements; for consideration of physiological aspects of isokinetic dynamometry, such as muscular adaptations with training and relationships with other physiological measurements, see for example Brown, 2000.

MECHANICAL BASIS OF ISOKINETIC DYNAMOMETRY MEASUREMENTS

An isokinetic dynamometer is a rotational device with a fixed axis of rotation that allows rotation with a constant angular velocity that is user selected. Figure 6.2 is a simplified schematic diagram of the basic components and operation of a typical isokinetic dynamometer. The user applies a force on the input arm as shown in Figure 6.2. This causes its rotation because it creates a moment, which is the product of the force applied on the input arm by the limb segment and its moment arm (shortest distance from the axis of rotation). The instantaneous angular velocity is monitored continuously and the braking mechanism is engaged accordingly, so that the required level of angular velocity is kept constant. The input arm is allowed to accelerate or decelerate if the instantaneous velocity is lower or higher than the pre-set target angular velocity, respectively. This represents a closed feedback loop mechanism with the actual (instantaneous) angular velocity as the controlled variable. Figure 6.3 describes the main steps in a typical feedback control loop in isokinetic machines.

The user selects the angular velocity required for the test (pre-set target velocity). Once the input arm starts rotating under the influence of an external moment (applied by the attached limb segment), the angular velocity sensor

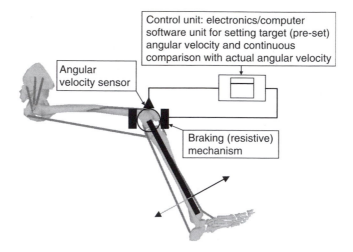

Figure 6.2   Schematic simplified diagram of the main components of an isokinetic dynamometer

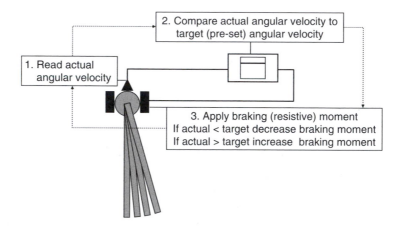

Figure 6.3   Schematic simplified diagram of the feedback loop for the control of the angular velocity by adjusting the resistive moment applied by the braking mechanism of the dynamometer. The resistive moment exerted against the limb depends on whether the actual angular velocity of the input arm is higher or lower compared to the user selected target (pre-set) angular velocity

registers the actual angular velocity of the input arm and this is compared with the required pre-set target velocity. If the actual velocity is lower than the required test velocity the controller signals the braking mechanism to reduce or maintain the resistance (braking) applied, so that the input arm can accelerate and increase the velocity further. If the actual velocity exceeds the pre-set target then the controller signals the braking mechanism to increase resistance, so that the input arm is decelerated and the actual velocity reduced. This feedback loop and control of the actual velocity is very fast and is repeated typically about 1,000 times per second or more, so effectively the angular velocity of the rotating arm is kept almost constant. It is not possible to have a completely constant velocity because the velocity control mechanism is always trying to 'catch-up' with the actual velocity of the input arm. However, because the control loop is repeated with such a high frequency ($\geqslant 1,000\,\text{Hz}$), the actual velocity is kept practically constant, at the level of the pre-set target velocity. From the above description it is evident that the isokinetic dynamometer provides the resistive moment required to maintain a constant angular velocity. The resistive mechanism depends on the type of isokinetic dynamometer; it could be based on hydraulics, electromechanical (motors) or a combination of the two types of components.

The resistive moment exerted by the braking mechanism, or the equivalent moment applied on the input arm by the segment, is provided as the main dynamometer system output together with the angular position of the input arm, usually via a dedicated computer system or analogue display devices on the dynamometer. However, what is required for the quantification of dynamic muscle strength is the actual joint moment applied by the muscles around the joint axis of rotation. It is very important to understand how this isokinetic dynamometer moment output is related to the joint moment because this has significant implications for the estimation of the joint moment and the interpretation of the isokinetic dynamometer data in general. The angular motion of the input arm around the fixed axis of rotation is governed by the same equation of planar motion for rotation (see equation 6.1 previously), so in a free body diagram of the dynamometer input arm for a knee extension test (Figure 6.4, left panel):

$$M_S - M_D - M_{GD} = I_D \cdot \alpha_D$$

where:

$\quad M_S$:   The moment of the segment force F_S around the axis of rotation of the dynamometer

$\quad M_D$:   The resistive moment exerted by the dynamometer

$\quad M_{GD}$:   The moment of the gravitational force F_{GD}

$\quad I_D$:   The moment of inertia of the dynamometer input arm

$\quad \alpha_D$:   The angular acceleration of the dynamometer input arm

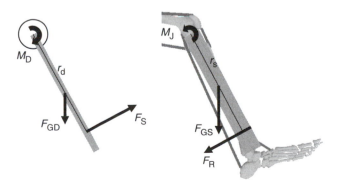

Figure 6.4 Free body diagrams of the dynamometer input arm (left) and the segment (right) for a knee extension test. Muscle strength is assessed by estimating the joint moment M_J from the dynamometer measured moment M_D

Assuming that the gravitational moment M_{GD} is measured and that the rotation is performed at an approximately constant velocity ($\alpha_D \approx 0$), then based on the above equation M_S can be calculated from M_D. So by monitoring M_D from the dynamometer during the constant velocity period we have effectively a measure of the M_S moment applied by the segment on the input arm and causing its rotation.

The angular motion of the segment around the joint axis of rotation is governed by the same equation of planar motion for rotation (see equation 6.1) so in a free body diagram of the segment (Figure 6.4, right panel):

$$M_J - M_R - M_{GS} = I_S \cdot \alpha_S$$

where:

M_J: The joint moment exerted mainly by the active muscle groups spanning the joint

M_R: The moment of the dynamometer resistive force F_R around the axis of rotation of the joint

M_{GS}:   The moment of the gravitational force F_{GS}

I_S: The moment of inertia of the limb segment

α_S: The angular acceleration of the limb segment

Assuming that M_{GS} is also measured and accounted for, and that the rotation is performed at an approximately constant velocity ($\alpha_S \approx 0$), then M_J can be calculated from M_R. Given that M_R is equal and opposite to M_S (since F_S and F_R are action and reaction and $r_d = r_s$) and M_S can be derived from M_D, we can then quantify M_J from M_D given the above gravity moment compensation and constant velocity assumptions. Surprisingly perhaps, the angular velocity, although measured and controlled, is not usually an output variable in most of the standard dynamometer software systems. This creates a number of important practical problems that affect the validity of measurements. As discussed above, there is a very important prerequisite for the joint moment M_J to be quantified from the dynamometer moment M_D: that the angular velocity is constant ($\alpha_D = \alpha_S = 0$), that is, the movement is isokinetic. If the input arm is accelerating or decelerating, then M_D is not equal to M_J and the angular acceleration must be measured (with video or accelerometers for example), but even then, the adjusted M_D could be at a velocity that is not equal to the pre-set target velocity. This has significant implications for the validity of the joint moment measurements and is discussed in detail in the Processing and Analysing Data section later.

The dynamometer moment M_D, corrected for gravitational and inertial effects, represents the two–dimensional component of the three–dimensional joint force and moment projected onto the plane of motion of the input arm around the fixed axis of rotation of the dynamometer (Kaufman et al., 1995). This is the sum of the moments exerted mainly by the various agonistic and antagonistic muscle groups and the ligaments around the different axes of rotation of the joint (e.g. extension–flexion, internal–external rotation, adduction–abduction). Although the dynamometer is designed to assess isolated joint motion around one of these axes during a particular test, these joint axes are affected by the moments at the joint. They also do not coincide with the fixed axis of rotation of the dynamometer throughout the range of motion, even after careful positioning and stabilisation of the subject. Movements around these axes are also interrelated. These joint-dynamometer axes misalignment problems will be discussed in detail later. It is also evident from the above that the recorded dynamometer moment is not to be confused with the moment of the muscle groups or individual muscles. Approximate estimation of the many individual muscle and ligament forces acting around joints during isokinetic testing is only possible using appropriate reduction or optimisation techniques for the distribution of the recorded moment to the individual force producing structures (Kaufman *et al.*, 1991). Some important problems and limitations with these techniques are discussed in relevant reviews (e.g. Tsirakos *et al.*, 1997). It follows that moment–velocity or moment–position relationships from the dynamometer measurements refer to the joint in general. They must not be confused with the force–velocity or force–length relationships of isolated muscles or a muscle group, even if that group is the most dominant and active during the movement.

Torque and moment definitions

Torque and moment (or moment of force more precisely) are both terms that are used to express the rotational effect of forces applied around an axis of rotation. They are normally used interchangeably in physics and in the isokinetic dynamometry literature; this quite often creates some confusion amongst readers and users of isokinetics. Mechanically they usually describe different force application situations relative to the long structural axis of a segment (see Figures 6.5 and 6.6). Both terms are appropriate depending on whether we consider the structural effects of the force on the input arm (bending moment) or the twisting effect on the central rod of the dynamometer (twisting moment or torque).

Because we are concerned with the moment applied on the input arm by the attached segment and the joint moment, the more appropriate term for this purpose and the one that will be used throughout this chapter is moment

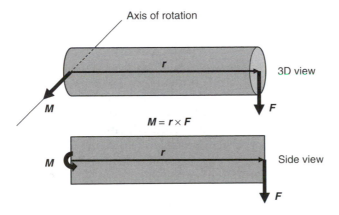

Figure 6.5 The definition of a moment (bending moment). Force vector and moment are perpendicular to the long structural axis

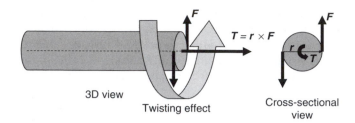

Figure 6.6 The definition of a torque (twisting moment) and the twisting effect. The axis of rotation is aligned with the long structural axis and the force pair is causing the torque. The torque vector is in line with the long structural axis and the axis of rotation

(measured in Nm or normalised to body mass as $Nm\,kg^{-1}$). Reference to torque will be made only when specifically referring to the twisting of the dynamometer central rod.

Main factors affecting isokinetic measurements

There are a number of factors affecting the quality and the validity of isokinetic measurements, so it is important to consider the following when using isokinetic dynamometers.

Angular velocity

An isokinetic dynamometer provides a record of the moment exerted through-out the movement and this is presented to the user on line (in real-time) or in digital format via the dedicated data analysis and presentation software, if storage and further processing is required. During an isokinetic test, the angular velocity of the input arm and segment increases from a stationary position (angular velocity is $0\ rad\,s^{-1}$) at the start of the movement to the target pre-set value, it is then maintained (approximately) constant by the velocity control mechanism, assuming that the person is able to apply the necessary moment to accelerate to the level of the pre-set velocity, and then decreases back to zero at the end of the range of motion (ROM). There is always an acceleration phase, followed by the constant angular velocity or isokinetic phase (angular acceleration ≈ 0) and then the deceleration phase. The relative duration of these three phases depends on the level of the pre-set target velocity, the ROM and the capabilities of the person and any preactivation of the muscles before the start of the movement. A number of studies have shown that the duration of the constant velocity (isokinetic) phase is reduced with increasing angular velocity tests, as expected. During very high angular velocity tests, the constant velocity or isokinetic phase is very limited (or nonexistent in very weak participants) and the majority of the ROM comprises of acceleration and deceleration. It is important to understand that although there is a moment output throughout the three phases, only the moment during the constant velocity (isokinetic) phase should be considered and used for analysis and assessment of dynamic strength.

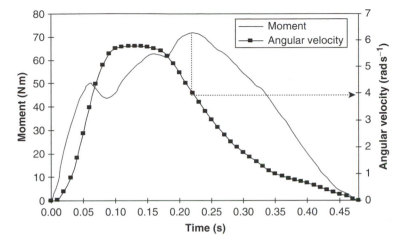

Figure 6.7 Moment and angular velocity during a knee extension test with the pre-set target velocity set at 5.23 rad s⁻¹ (300 deg s⁻¹). Notice that the maximum moment was recorded when the angular velocity was just under 4 rad s⁻¹ during the deceleration (non-isokinetic) period

The moment data during the acceleration and deceleration phases should be discarded because, even if corrected for inertial effects, they are not recorded and produced at the required target velocity and in isokinetic conditions. This, however, requires checking of the angular velocity over the same timeframe as the moment output so that the instantaneous angular velocity for each moment value is known. Figure 6.7 is such an example of moment – time and angular velocity – time displayed together to allow a simple check of the moment data portion that was recorded at isokinetic (constant angular velocity) conditions.

Despite the importance of this check, the moment and angular velocity are not very often displayed together in the standard dedicated computer software of most isokinetic machines, even though the angular velocity is monitored and recorded in all isokinetic systems. If this option is not available in the dedicated computer software then the user must perform this check independently. This can be done in a number of ways depending on the dynamometer and software used. For example, the CYBEX Norm model has an auxiliary interface card that can be installed separately and it allows access to the analogue data output of torque, angular position, angular velocity and direction of movement. The user can sample these analogue signals using a standard analogue to digital (A/D) conversion system and display them together in a separate computer system used for data collection. The dedicated computer-software system is still required for dynamometer set-up and control. In more recent software updates for the CYBEX range of dynamometers (HUMAC system) there are enhanced options for exporting all data after collection, including angular velocity. In other systems, such as the BIODEX dynamometer, the angular velocity signal is sampled and is also available for exporting via the standard software. Further details of the sampling resolution and accuracy characteristics of these hardware and software components are provided in the following section on Isokinetic Equipment Considerations.

The angular velocity values will contain some noise (from the A/D conversion and/or the differentiation of the angular position data if the angular velocity is not recorded directly). Furthermore, as explained earlier, the velocity control mechanism will always have some very small time delay ('trailing behind') so it is not possible to have a numerically exact constant value even in the constant angular velocity (isokinetic) period. For these reasons the angular velocity data require some filtering (see Chapter 7) and the isokinetic phase must then be determined with a reasonable limit for the filtered angular velocity fluctuation. This is normally between 5 and 10 per cent of the target pre-set value to accommodate different velocity control mechanisms and noise levels.

If an isokinetic dynamometer is used for research or any kind of dynamic strength assessment, especially when high joint angular velocities are used (>3–$4\,\mathrm{rad\,s^{-1}}$), then it is essential to have access to the digital or analogue angular velocity signal through the standard or any available auxiliary output. Simultaneous checking of the moment and the corresponding angular velocity over time is necessary to identify the isokinetic phase in high pre-set angular velocities tests and avoid gross errors in the assessment of joint moment and dynamic strength. This is not required, or is not as critical, at slower velocity tests.

The operation of the dynamometer mechanism during the initial acceleration period in concentric tests is another important mechanical problem. In some isokinetic dynamometers, the body segment is allowed to accelerate up to the level of the pre-set angular velocity without much resistance. In this case the dynamometer moment will be very close to zero for a brief initial period but obviously there will be a joint moment accelerating the system. When the segment is approaching the pre-set target velocity, the resistive mechanism is suddenly activated and required to apply a large moment to prevent further acceleration of the segment. This initial resistive moment appears as a prominent overshoot in the dynamometer moment recording ('torque overshoot') and leads to a sudden impact and deceleration of the input arm and body segment. Depending on the pre-set velocity and the capabilities of the participant, this overshoot could be much higher than the maximum moment of the joint at that position. This could lead to overloading and possible injury, especially with repeated impacts. Modern dynamometers apply some resistive moment during the acceleration phase, irrespective of the actual angular velocity magnitude, and this helps to avoid the need for a sudden application of a large resistive moment as the segment approaches the pre-set velocity target. This response of the braking mechanism and the amount of resistive moment applied at the beginning of the movement, until the pre-set velocity is reached, is normally adjustable and is described as 'cushioning'. See the section on Processing and Analysing Data for the effects of these options on the isokinetic parameters.

Gravitational moment

The total moment applied around the dynamometer axis and recorded by the torque transducer is the result of the effect of all the moments applied on the

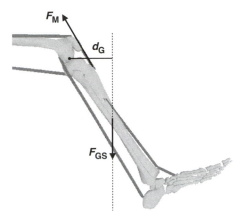

Figure 6.8 Gravitational moment due to the weight of the segment (F_{GS}) acting with a moment arm d_G around the axis of rotation of the joint. Since the gravitational force is constant, the gravitational moment will depend on d_G and will be maximum at full extension and zero with the segment in the vertical position (90° of knee flexion in this example)

input arm, including the gravitational moments due to the weight of the input arm itself and the attached segment. For example, if the input arm is locked (for isometric testing) in the horizontal position with the attached limb segment relaxed, there will still be a flexion moment recorded due to the moments caused by the weights of the input arm and the limb segment. The total gravitational moment will be a function of the cosine of the input arm angle, being maximum in the horizontal position (0°) and zero in the vertical position (90°) – see Figure 6.8.

Most isokinetic systems include an automated gravity moment correction procedure as part of the dedicated software system. This involves the measurement of the total gravitational moment during a passive weighing of the segment either throughout the range of motion or at a mid-range position. The moment recorded during the test is then adjusted by either subtracting or adding (depending on the direction of the input arm movement) the measured or calculated moment due to gravity at the different positions.

It is important to point out that the gravitational effect is an issue only for movements in the vertical plane. If it is technically possible for the dynamometer main unit to be tilted so that its axis of rotation was vertical and the segment plane of motion was horizontal (e.g. elbow flexion–extension with the lower arm attached to the input arm of the dynamometer with the upper arm abducted 90° and horizontal) then the gravitational moments would not affect the moments recorded by the dynamometer.

Axes of rotation alignment

Isokinetic dynamometers are designed to measure the moment applied around their fixed axis of rotation. Therefore, to exert the maximum rotational effect

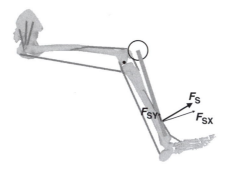

Figure 6.9 Effects of misalignment of axes of rotation. The axes of rotation of the segment and dynamometer input arm are not aligned and, in this case, the long axes of the segment and input arm are not parallel either. Because the segment attachment pad rotates freely and is rigidly attached to the segment, the force applied by the segment (F_S) is perpendicular to its long axis but not perpendicular to the dynamometer input arm. As a result, only a component (F_{SX}) of the applied force F_s is producing a moment around the axis of rotation of the dynamometer

(moment) possible, the force applied must be perpendicular to the long axis of the input arm. If an external force is applied by the segment at an angle other than 90° to the input arm then only the perpendicular component will be generating a moment (Figure 6.9). In the most extreme case for example, if the external force is applied along the long axis of the input arm, then there will be no moment generated or recorded since the force will be acting through the axis of rotation of the dynamometer (moment arm = 0).

It was shown earlier in this section using the free body diagrams of the segment and the input arm, that one of the necessary conditions for using M_D from the dynamometer to quantify the joint moment M_J is that $M_S = M_R$ (see Figure 6.4). Since by definition F_R is equal and opposite to F_S (action–reaction) then the moment arms of these two forces (r_s and r_d) must also be equal.

The only way for $r_s = r_d$ is for the axes of rotation of the segment and the dynamometer to be aligned. If the joint axis of rotation is not in alignment with the dynamometer axis then r_s will be different to r_d and therefore $M_S \neq M_R \Rightarrow M_J \neq M_D$ so we will not be able to quantify the joint moment from the dynamometer moment.

For example, let us assume that the long axes of the segment and the input arm overlap on the sagittal plane, but the joint axis of rotation is located 2 cm above the dynamometer axis of rotation and the input arm is attached 30 cm from the joint axis so that $r_s = 0.3$ m but $r_d = 0.28$ m (Figure 6.10).

If the joint moment exerted was known and was $M_J = 270$ N m then the force F_S applied to the input arm and its reaction applied on the segment F_R will be $F_S = F_R = 900$ N: $M_J = M_R = 900 \times 0.3 = 270$ N m.

The 900 N applied on the input arm of the dynamometer, 28 cm from its fixed axis of rotation will be generating a moment $M_S = 900 \times 0.28 = 252$ N m and this will be registered by the dynamometer. So this 2 cm error in the alignment of the axes of rotation will be causing an error of 18 N m (6.6 per cent) in the measurement of joint moments: $((270 - 252) / 272) \times 100$.

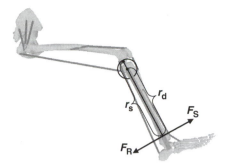

Figure 6.10   An example of dynamometer and joint axis of rotation misalignment. In this case, the long axes of the segment and input arm are parallel (coincide in 2D) so the force applied by the segment F_S is perpendicular to the input arm but the moment arms of the forces F_S and F_R relative to the dynamometer ($r_d = 0.28$ m) and joint ($r_s = 0.3$ m) axis of rotation, respectively, are different. As a result, the joint moment (M_J) and the dynamometer recorded moment (M_D) are also different. (Gravitational forces are ignored in this example)

In general if $r_d \neq r_s$ then (ignoring gravitational and inertial forces)

$$M_J = F_R r_s \text{ and } F_R = M_J/r_s$$
$$M_D = F_S r_d \text{ and } F_S = M_D/r_d$$

and since $F_R = F_S$ then $M_J/r_s = M_D/r_d$ and

$$M_J = M_D(r_s/r_d)$$

In general then, if the moment arms of the segment and the dynamometer are different because of the misalignment of joint and dynamometer axes of rotation, then the dynamometer moment M_D must be corrected by multiplying it with the ratio of the moment arms (r_s/r_d). This is the only way to measure the joint moment accurately. Although the moment arm of the input arm force does not change (r_d is a constant), the moment arm of the segment will be changing based on the position of the joint centre (axis of rotation) throughout the motion. In the knee, for example, a number of studies have examined the error caused by the misalignment of the axes of rotation of the joint and the dynamometer during contraction. Herzog, 1988, examined a single participant using a Cybex II dynamometer and a two-dimensional kinematic analysis system filming at a frequency of 50 Hz. He reported that the maximum differences between the actual knee joint moment and the recorded moment during isometric and isokinetic knee extension trials at 120 and 240 deg s^{-1} were 1.5, 1.3 and 2.1 per cent, respectively. Kaufman *et al.*, 1995, quantified the errors associated with the misalignment of the knee joint axis and the dynamometer axis of rotation during isokinetic (60 and 180 deg s^{-1}) knee extensions on five normal participants. They also used a Cybex II isokinetic dynamometer and they measured the three-dimensional kinematics of the leg using a tri-axial electrogoniometer. They found that the average differences between the actual and recorded knee joint moments were 10 and 13 per cent during isokinetic knee extensions at 60 and 180 deg s^{-1}, respectively.

More recently, Arampatzis *et al.*, 2004, determined the differences between the actual moment and the moment measured by dynamometry at the knee joint on 27 athletes during isometric knee extension. A Biodex dynamometer was used for the quantification of joint moments and a Vicon system with eight cameras operating at 120 Hz was used for recording three-dimensional kinematic data of the leg. They reported differences between the dynamometer and the actual joint moment ranging from 0.33–17 per cent (average 7.3 per cent).

It must be emphasised that the positioning and stabilisation of the participants in all of the above studies were performed following the manufacturer's recommendations, using the standard belts, straps and other mechanical restraints supplied. Furthermore, the reported joint moment errors were totally inconsistent between participants and testing sessions and depended on the stabilisation of the participant, the movement of the isolated and moving segments relative to the dynamometer due to the compliance of the soft tissue and the dynamometer components, such as the seat and input arm padding. Other factors contributing to the random nature of the errors present in the joint moment measurement are, the initial alignment of the axes, the mode and intensity of contraction and the range of motion.

It is important to understand that there will always be a misalignment of the axes because: (a) joints do not have fixed axes of rotation and the changing instantaneous joint axis cannot be aligned with a fixed axis (dynamometer) throughout the ROM and (b) no matter how carefully the joint axis is aligned with the dynamometer axis in a specific position there will always be some movement of the segment relative to the input arm during the movement. Therefore, there will always be some change of the segment moment arm due to the compliance and compression of soft tissues (muscles, subcutaneous fat etc) and the dynamometer components (chair and input arm attachment padding). The wide range of the joint moment errors reported (0.33–17 per cent by Arampatzis *et al.*, 2004) within the same group of participants tested by the same investigators using standardised and recommended procedures for a relatively simple and highly constrained contraction mode (isometric) shows the scale of the problem and the important implications if this error is not minimised during the data collection procedures, or corrected afterwards.

Adjacent joints' position and bi-articular muscle length effects

Isokinetic dynamometry involves single joint testing so only the tested joint is allowed to move over its range of motion. All the other joints should be fixed and the segments stabilised to avoid extraneous movement and possible contributions. However, when bi-articular muscles are involved and these span the tested joint, it is important to consider carefully, record and standardise the position of the adjacent joints spanned by the bi-articular muscles. This is because the muscle force and, as a result, its contribution to the joint moment depends on the length of the muscles according to the force–length relationship as well as the velocity and mode of action as explained previously. For example, hip angle must be standardised during knee extension to avoid variations in the length of the rectus femoris, as it has been shown that the knee extension moment is different between supine and seated positions (e.g. Pavol and Grabiner, 2000; Maffiuletti and Lepers, 2003). Similarly, during a knee flexion test on the dynamometer, the length of the hamstrings will also be affected by the hip angle and chair position. Furthermore, the position of the ankle (plantarflexion or dorsiflexion) will affect the length of the bi-articular gastrocnemius, which is a muscle that can also contribute to knee flexion moment under sufficient length conditions. It has been shown, for example, that knee flexion moment is higher with the knee flexion test performed with the ankle in dorsiflexion (longer gastrocnemius length) compared to knee flexion with the ankle in full plantarflexion (Croce *et al.*, 2000). So in this case not only the angle of the hip joint, but also the ankle joint angle, should be standardised and controlled.

ISOKINETIC EQUIPMENT CONSIDERATIONS

This section describes the main considerations when choosing an isokinetic device. The isokinetic equipment market has been quite volatile in recent years because of the availability of an increasing number of different machines from established and new manufacturers and the saturated market for isokinetic equipment in rehabilitation centres, universities and other clinical research facilities. As a result, a number of manufacturers have ceased trading altogether or they have closed down the isokinetic equipment part of the business and no further support or products are offered. However, their machines are still used and it may be possible to buy second-hand machines from previous users (e.g. Lido, MERAC, AKRON, Technogym Rev 9000). This chapter will only consider isokinetic equipment, which, at the time of writing, is still available from authorised companies that can offer service and maintenance or repair support.

Isokinetic hardware and software

All the modern available isokinetic dynamometers use electromechanical components for the control of the angular velocity of the input arm. Hydraulic based systems are no longer available, with the exception of used KinCom models that are based on a combination of electromechanical and hydraulic components or other used hydraulic-based systems such as the AKRON. Older models (e.g. Cybex II) had a passive resistive mechanism and resistance was developed only as a reaction to the applied joint moment. This mechanism allowed only concentric muscle action. The modern electromechanical dynamometers (e.g. Biodex, CON-TREX, Cybex NORM, IsoMed 2000) have active mechanisms as well as the standard passive operation in the concentric mode. These dynamometers are capable of driving the input arm at a pre-set angular velocity irrespective of the moment applied by the person being tested. This allows eccentric muscle action at constant angular velocities. The operation of the resistive mechanism, and the control of the angular velocity and acceleration in these systems, requires the use of appropriate dedicated computer systems. However, there are considerable differences in the techniques implemented in the software of various dynamometers. These differences concern the collection and processing of moment data and the calculation of different mechanical variables, such as the gravitational moment, joint moment, angular velocity of motion, and moment developed in the initial acceleration period. For these reasons, the software-computer system features, user-friendliness and any options must all be examined in detail to ensure that they are the best for the intended use of the equipment (research, rehabilitation, teaching, or combination of uses). Some dynamometers offer control via both the computer system and an analogue or digital control panel (e.g. Biodex) and this can be very useful, for example, in teaching/demonstrating applications.

Angular velocities range and moment limits

The range of angular velocities available under concentric and eccentric modes and the respective maximum moment limits are some of the most important features in an isokinetic dynamometer. Table 6.1 summarises these characteristics in some of the most popular commercially available isokinetic dynamometers.

Isokinetic data resolution and accuracy considerations

The quality, reliability and hysterisis characteristics of the modern transducers used in the new generation of isokinetic dynamometers are very good. The accuracy of the torque, angle and angular velocity data has improved considerably in modern systems and typical values in different machines range

Table 6.1 Summary of the range or limits of angular velocities and moments under concentric and eccentric modes for the most popular commercially available isokinetic dynamometers, including manufacturer website information

Dynamometer	Angular velocity (rad s^{-1})		Moment limits (N m)	
	C	E	C	E
Biodex www.biodex.com	0.5–8	0.1–2.6	610	410
CON-TREX www.con-trex.ch	8.7	8.7	720	720
Cybex Norm www.csmisolutions.com	0.1–8.7	0.1–5.2	680	680
IsoMed 2000 www.isomed2000.de	7.8–9.7		500–750	
KinCom 500H www.kincom.com	0.02–4.4	0.02–4.4	800*	800*

Notes
C: concentric; E: eccentric. *Values obtained by assuming a moment arm of 0.4 m.

from ± 0.25 to ± 1 per cent of full scale for torque and less than about 0.3 per cent of full scale for angle or from less than $\pm 0.1°$ to $\pm 1°$. One of the most important considerations is access to the analogue or digital data of angle, torque and angular velocity, especially when the isokinetic dynamometer is used for research purposes. Older systems provided digital data with limited sampling rates (100–120 Hz) and access to the analogue data was only possible with optional accessory components at an extra cost. For example it is possible to fit an auxiliary interface board to the later Cybex machines (e.g. NORM) that provides access to the analogue signals of torque, angular position, velocity and direction of movement. The analogue output can then be sampled using an A/D converter completely independently of the dedicated software/computer with a higher, user-determined sampling frequency. This is essential for research applications. Modern isokinetic systems (e.g. Biodex System 3, CON-TREX, IsoMed 2000) include 12- or 16-bit A/D converters resulting in a resolution of $\sim \pm 0.0244$ per cent of full scale. Very high sampling rates of up to 4000 Hz or 5000 Hz further means that the resolution and accuracy of the digital data provided by the standard computer systems in these modern machines are quite adequate for research purposes.

Isokinetic equipment rigidity and space considerations

The overall strength and rigidity of the dynamometer and the stiffness of all the components are also very important considerations, especially when testing very strong athletes such as sprinters, rugby players, power lifters etc. For example, it is unfortunately very common in older machines for the main unit to twist from its base where it is attached on the frame of the dynamometer when very strong athletes apply high moments, resulting in an unsafe situation and certainly invalid measurements. Modern dynamometers are heavier and more rigid with stronger and better supporting frames for the chair and main unit, but, ideally, the user must try a new machine with a sample of the likely population that they will be using in their work. The overall mass of isokinetic dynamometers is normally in the range of 500–700 kg and they typically require a minimum space of 6–7 m^2 for standard operation.

ISOKINETIC EXPERIMENTAL AND DATA COLLECTION PROCEDURES

The following factors can affect the overall quality of isokinetic data and have significant implications for assessment of joint function. They need to be considered in detail when setting up an isokinetic device for data collection.

Calibration

Moment calibration can be performed using gravitational loading under static or slow velocity conditions. Most manufacturers provide accurate calibration weights; to calibrate a large range of moments, a range of weights should be used. Accurate goniometers can be used to calibrate angular position. Several dynamometers also include a self-calibration mechanism for checking and adjusting the zero baseline or factory calibration of the torque transducer. Full calibration of the measurement system (moment and angle transducers) should be performed at the manufacturer recommended intervals or periodically, depending on usage, and recorded on a technical calibration log. Checking of the complete measurement and recording system (including interface boards, any amplifiers and analogue-to-digital converter) must be performed before each measurement session irrespective of the type of dynamometer used.

Familiarisation instructions

Constant angular velocity movements are rarely performed during exercise or sports activities; it is therefore important to familiarise the subjects with this mode of joint action before the test. The complete range of the angular velocities to be used in the test must be included in the familiarisation session. Standardised instructions should be given, explaining that isokinetic testing involves variable resistance at a constant velocity and stressing the importance of maximum muscular effort during the tests. The maintenance of maximum effort, throughout the range of movement, by both muscle groups during reciprocal movements, such as knee extension–flexion, must be specifically emphasised. Failure to include familiarisation with this mode of joint function may have serious effects on the reliability of measurements.

Participant positioning

The person being tested should be stabilised to ensure that the recorded moment is generated by the examined joint muscles only, without any contribution from other actions. During a typical single segment movement, such as knee extension–flexion, the opposite leg, the waist, torso and the arms should be stabilised with appropriate belts or harnesses, usually provided by the manufacturers of the dynamometer. The examined body segment should be securely fastened to the input arm of the dynamometer to avoid moment overshoots and to prevent injury from impacts between the limb and the input arm. If bi-articular muscles are involved then the angles of the adjacent joints should be considered carefully and must be standardised and controlled during the test to avoid bi-articular muscle contribution errors (see earlier discussion). It is particularly important if a retest is performed to have a detailed record of all the test settings to ensure high repeatability and accurate conclusions.

The axis of rotation of the dynamometer must be aligned carefully with the joint axis to minimise axes misalignment errors. Although the instantaneous axis of rotation of a joint is difficult to establish visually and varies in dynamic conditions, an approximation using relevant anatomical landmarks is essential. For example, the most prominent point on the lateral epicondyle of the femur as palpated externally on the lateral surface of the knee joint or the most prominent point on the lateral malleolus for the ankle. A laser pointing device, or some other alignment tool, can be used to improve the alignment of the dynamometer axis with the anatomical landmark, or other point that the joint axis of rotation is assumed to pass through. Given that there is a large change in joint position and angle between rest and contraction (e.g. Arampatzis *et al.*, 2004; 2005), it is necessary to align the axes during submaximal or maximal contraction and not with the segment at rest. In order to minimise further the axes misalignment error in specific parameters such as the maximum joint moment, the active alignment (under maximal or submaximal contraction conditions) should be performed near the joint position where the maximum joint moment is expected or at the joint angle where any angle-specific moment will be measured.

Range of motion

The range of movement must be set according to the physiological limits of the joint and activated muscle group and any inhibiting injuries; it must also be standardised and controlled. Standardisation of the range of movement also facilitates data analysis, for example integration of the moment with respect to angular displacement to calculate mechanical work. The angular velocity of the movement should be set according to the objectives of the test and the muscular capabilities of those being tested. During fast velocity testing ($>3.1\,\mathrm{rad\,s^{-1}}$) it must be ensured that the person can achieve the pre-set velocity within the range of joint movement. The duration of the isokinetic (constant velocity) phase of the movement decreases as the test speed is increased, as more time is required to reach higher pre-set velocities and to decelerate at the end of the movement. This is important, as the dynamometer moment in concentric conditions is not equal to the joint moment if the pre-set velocity is not attained and kept constant, as explained earlier.

Preloading

Preloading of the muscles, using electrical stimulation or manual resistance before the release of the isokinetic mechanism, can be used to facilitate the development of faster joint velocities over limited ranges of movement.

Gravity correction

Most computerised dynamometers include gravity correction as part of the experimental protocol; this correction must be performed before each test of joint function to minimise measurement errors. If a computerised procedure is not available, a simple method for gravity correction should be used. One method involves the recording of the gravitational moment generated by the weight of the segment and lever arm falling passively against the resistance of the dynamometer, at a specific angular position within the range of movement. The gravitational moment at different angular positions is then calculated as a function of the gravitational moment at the measurement position and joint angle. This procedure must be performed at the minimum angular velocity or under isometric conditions. The limb must be relaxed and the muscle groups involved, both agonists and antagonists, must not be close to their maximum length, to avoid unwanted contributions from the elastic components. In practice, it is suggested that several trials should be performed to ensure complete muscular relaxation during this measurement. It has been shown, however, that this method gives an overestimation of the actual gravitational moment of the segment, because of the elastic effects of the musculotendinous unit and incomplete relaxation (Kellis and Baltzopoulos, 1996). Estimation of the gravitational moment from anthropometric data has been found to be a more accurate gravity correction method; it is therefore suggested that this method may be a useful alternative to the passive fall method. The gravitational moment at different angular positions is then added to the dynamometer moment produced by muscle groups opposed by gravity, for example the quadriceps femoris in a knee extension–flexion movement in the sagittal plane (see Figure 6.4 and related equations). For muscle groups facilitated by gravity, such as the hamstrings, the gravitational moment is subtracted from the recorded moment.

Performance feedback

Visual feedback of joint moment data during isokinetic testing has a significant effect on the maximum moment. The magnitude of this effect depends on the angular velocity of movement. It is therefore important to provide visual feedback of the muscular performance during the test, particularly during maximum moment assessment at slow angular velocities. The real-time display of the moment output on a computer monitor, or other display device, can be used for visual feedback. It is important to give detailed instructions on the interpretation of the different sources of visual feedback and the performance target. Verbal motivation for maximum effort must be given in the form of standardised and consistent instructions/encouragement.

Control and standardisation of experimental procedures

Differences in the experimental factors described in this section can significantly affect moment measurements. Different isokinetic dynamometers also use different settings and testing procedures. It is evident from the above, that testing of the same person on different machines will most likely produce different results, because of biological and mechanical variations. Differences in data processing from different software applications introduce further discrepancies into the assessment of joint function. Joint function measurements are therefore specific to the dynamometer, the procedures and the data processing techniques used. Comparison of results from different dynamometers, even from the same person, is not possible. For these reasons, it is essential to standardise and report (see Reporting an Isokinetic Study section) the relevant details of the experimental procedures and data processing; it is particularly important to use exactly the same settings in test–retest experiments.

In summary:

- Calibrate dynamometer or check accuracy of data output.
- Familiarise participants and give clear and standardised, consistent instructions.
- Take particular care during eccentric tests and when testing children, or weak or injured/operated subjects.
- Stabilise and control adjacent joints when bi-articular muscles are involved.
- Stabilise segments and reduce extraneous movement.
- Align axes of rotation:
  o accurately
  o under maximal contraction conditions
  o near the position of expected maximum joint moment.
- Monitor angular velocity independently.

PROCESSING, ANALYSING AND PRESENTING ISOKINETIC DATA

Angular velocity monitoring and isokinetic data processing

To overcome measurement errors resulting from the overshoot in the moment recordings, analogue electrical filters have been used to dampen the overshoot and smooth the signal. Different cut-off frequencies (damping settings) have been suggested, depending on the angular velocity of the movement and the testing conditions. These electrical filters introduce a phase shift into the moment-time signal; the overshoot peak is reduced, and the filter also reduces the magnitude of the moment throughout the range of movement. The use of such filters must therefore be avoided, as it leads to significant distortion of the moment-angular position relationship that is the basis for the measurement of most isokinetic joint function parameters. Some isokinetic dynamometers (e.g. Biodex) apply a resistive moment from the start of the concentric movement, before the development of the pre-set velocity, just by sensing movement of the input arm. This reduces the acceleration rate and therefore the time required to attain the pre-set velocity is increased. However, the transition from acceleration to the pre-set constant angular velocity is smoother and no sudden resistive overshoot moment is required.

Only the isokinetic part of the movement should be considered and moment data must be analysed from the constant angular velocity part of the movement only (Figure 6.11), irrespective of the method used to control acceleration and its effects on movement recording. Although several dynamometers provide angular velocity data, it has been shown that these

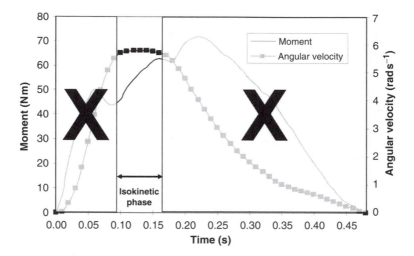

Figure 6.11 At high target velocities the isokinetic (constant angular velocity) movement is very limited or non-existent. In this test with the target velocity preset at $5.23\,\mathrm{rad\,s^{-1}}$ ($300\,\mathrm{deg\,s^{-1}}$), the isokinetic phase lasts only approximately $0.075\,\mathrm{s}$, and is only about 15 per cent of the total extension movement. Moment data outside this interval should be discarded because they do not occur in isokinetic (constant angular velocity) conditions and the actual angular velocity of movement is always slower than the required pre-set velocity

measurements may contain large errors, particularly during tests with a high pre-set angular velocity (Iossifidou and Baltzopoulos, 1998; 2000). It is therefore recommended that the user should independently calculate kinematic variables, such as the angular velocity and acceleration of the body segment, using the angular position time data provided by the dynamometer. This should only be done if the angular position has been calibrated before the test. The digital data contain errors (noise) mainly from the analogue-to-digital conversion; appropriate noise reduction techniques are therefore needed for the accurate measurement of kinematic variables. Several noise reduction and differentiation techniques (e.g. digital filters, spline functions and truncated Fourier series) that have been applied in other areas of biomechanics research (see Chapters 2 and 3) are appropriate.

Isokinetic parameters

Maximum moment

The maximum moment during an isokinetic movement is an indicator of the maximum muscular force applied in dynamic conditions (dynamic strength). Various testing protocols have been used for the assessment of this maximum moment; it is usually evaluated from three to six maximal repetitions and defined as the maximum single moment value measured during these repetitions. The average value of the maximum moments from several repetitions should not be used as an indication of the maximum joint moment. The maximum moment depends on the joint position at which it was recorded, as this position affects the force–length relationship of the active muscles. A maximum moment, calculated as the average of several maximum moment values recorded at different joint positions, is not an appropriate measure of muscle function, as it provides no information about the joint moment–position relationship. The average from several repetitions is only useful when the moment is recorded at a specific predetermined joint position in each repetition. In this case, however, the recorded moment at the predetermined position may not be the maximum moment for that repetition.

Reciprocal muscle group moment ratios

The reciprocal muscle group ratio is an indicator of joint balance; it is usually affected by age, sex and physical activity (Baltzopoulos and Brodie, 1989). The measurement of reciprocal muscle group ratios must be performed using gravity-corrected moment data to avoid errors in the assessment of muscle function.

Angle of maximum moment

The joint angular position is important in the assessment of muscle function because it provides information about the mechanical properties of the activated muscle groups. The maximum moment position is affected by the angular velocity of the movement; it tends to occur later in the range of movement with increasing velocity, and not at the mechanically optimal joint position. Furthermore, it is essential to check whether the maximum moment was recorded at a joint position in which the angular velocity was constant. Consequently, analysis of maximum moment data, irrespective of angular position, may lead to erroneous conclusions about muscle function.

Fatigue and endurance

Muscular endurance under isokinetic conditions is the ability of the activated muscle groups to sustain a movement with maximum effort at the pre-set angular velocity. It is usually assessed by computing a fatigue index. However, there is neither a standardised testing protocol for the assessment of muscular endurance nor an agreed definition of the fatigue index. It has been suggested that muscular endurance should be assessed: over 30 to 50 repetitions; up until the moment has fallen to 50 per cent of the maximum initial moment; or over a total duration of 30 to 60 s. The fatigue index can be expressed as a ratio between the maximum moment in the initial and final periods of the test. The mechanical work performed is a more representative measure of muscle function, because it is computed from the moment output throughout the range of movement. To compute the fatigue index from mechanical work measurements, however, the range of movement must be standardised and the moment data must be corrected for the effects of gravitational and inertial forces.

Acceleration related parameters

Some isokinetic parameters for the analysis of concentric muscle function during the initial part of the movement (such as joint moment development and time to maximum moment) have been based on dynamometer moment data during the acceleration period. It is evident from the description of the isokinetic measurement process that, in concentric conditions, the dynamometer moment during this initial acceleration period represents the resistive moment developed by the dynamometer and not the actual joint moment accelerating the system. Furthermore, the resistive dynamometer moment in concentric conditions is delayed until the pre-set velocity is attained by the moving limb and depends also on the response of the resistive mechanism in different types of dynamometers and any relevant settings used (e.g. cushioning, damping etc). Consequently, any conclusions about the mechanical properties of the muscle group, based on the dynamometer moment output during the initial acceleration period, are invalid. The joint moment during the acceleration and deceleration periods should not be used for any measurements (e.g. 'torque acceleration energy') and only the isokinetic phase moment should be analysed, as explained in the Angular Velocity Monitoring and Isokinetic Data Processing section.

REPORTING AN ISOKINETIC STUDY

Full details of the following should be included in the report of an isokinetic study:

- Isokinetic dynamometer make and type.
- Details of data acquisition: it is essential to report whether the standard software of the dynamometer or an independent system was used to sample the analogue signals. In this case the details of the sampling and A/D processes are necessary (sampling frequency, resolution and accuracy of moment and angular position measurements, etc.).
- Procedures followed for calibration and/or checking of measurements and gravity correction.
- Test settings (eccentric/concentric, range of movement, angular velocity, feedback type and method).
- Participant positioning: given the effects of axes misalignment, the method of axes alignment used must be described in detail. The angle of adjacent joints (e.g. hip and ankle joint position during knee tests) must also be reported.
- Isokinetic (constant angular velocity) phase determination: details of angular velocity monitoring method (dynamometer software or independent sampling) and determination of the constant velocity (isokinetic) phase. This can be omitted in slow velocity testing ($<180 \deg s^{-1}$) but it is essential in high velocity testing.

REFERENCES

Arampatzis, A., Karamanidis, K., De Monte, G., Stafilidis, S., Morey-Klapsing, G. and Bruggemann, G. P. (2004) 'Differences between measured and resultant joint moments during voluntary and artificially elicited isometric knee extension contractions', *Clinical Biomechanics*, 19(3): 277–283.

Arampatzis, A., Morey-Klapsing, G., Karamanidis, K., DeMonte, G., Stafilidis, S. and Bruggemann, G. P. (2005) 'Differences between measured and resultant joint moments during isometric contractions at the ankle joint', *Journal of Biomechanics*, 38(4): 885–892.

Baltzopoulos, V. and Brodie, D. A. (1989) 'Isokinetic dynamometry. Applications and limitations', *Sports Medicine*, 8(2): 101–116.

Brown L. E. (2000) *Isokinetics in Human Performance*, Champaign, IL: Human Kinetics.

Cabri, J. M. (1991) 'Isokinetic strength aspects of human joints and muscles', *Critical Reviews in Biomedical Engineering*, 19(2-3): 231–259.

Chan, K.-M., Maffulli, N., Korkia, P. and Li Raymond, C. T. (1996) *Principles and Practice of Isokinetics in Sports Medicine and Rehabilitation*, Hong Kong: Williams and Wilkins.

Croce, R. V., Miller, J. P. and St Pierre, P. (2000) 'Effect of ankle position fixation on peak torque and electromyographic activity of the knee flexors and extensors', *Electromyography and Clinical Neurophysiology*, 40(6): 365–373.

De Ste Croix, M., Deighan, M. and Armstrong, N. (2003) 'Assessment and interpretation of isokinetic muscle strength during growth and maturation', *Sports Medicine*, 33(10): 727–743.

Dvir, Z. (ed.) (2004) *Isokinetics: Muscle Testing, Interpretation and Clinical Applications*, 2nd edn, Edinburgh: Churchill Livingstone.

Gleeson, N. P. and Mercer, T. H. (1996) 'The utility of isokinetic dynamometry in the assessment of human muscle function', *Sports Medicine*, 21(1): 18–34.

Herzog, W. (1988) 'The relation between the resultant moments at a joint and the moments measured by an isokinetic dynamometer', *Journal of Biomechanics*, 21(1): 5–12.

Iossifidou, A. N. and Baltzopoulos, V. (1998) 'Inertial effects on the assessment of performance in isokinetic dynamometry', *International Journal of Sports Medicine*, 19(8): 567–573.

Iossifidou, A. N. and Baltzopoulos, V. (2000) 'Inertial effects on moment development during isokinetic concentric knee extension testing', *Journal of Orthopaedic and Sports Physical Therapy*, 30(6): 317–323; discussion: 324–317.

Kannus, P. (1994) 'Isokinetic evaluation of muscular performance: Implications for muscle testing and rehabilitation', *International Journal of Sports Medicine*, 15 Suppl 1, S11–18.

Kaufman, K. R., An, K. N. and Chao, E. Y. (1995) 'A comparison of intersegmental joint dynamics to isokinetic dynamometer measurements', *Journal of Biomechanics*, 28(10): 1243–1256.

Kaufman, K. R., An, K. N., Litchy, W. J., Morrey, B. F. and Chao, E. Y. (1991) 'Dynamic joint forces during knee isokinetic exercise', *American Journal of Sports Medicine*, 19(3): 305–316.

Kellis, E. and Baltzopoulos, V. (1995) 'Isokinetic eccentric exercise', *Sports Medicine*, 19(3): 202–222.

Kellis, E. and Baltzopoulos, V. (1996) 'Gravitational moment correction in isokinetic dynamometry using anthropometric data', *Medicine and Science in Sports and Exercise*, 28(7): 900–907.

King, M. A. and Yeadon, M. R. (2002) 'Determining subject-specific torque parameters for use in a torque-driven simulation model of dynamic jumping', *Journal of Applied Biomechanics*, 18(3): 207–217.

Maffiuletti, N. A. and Lepers, R. (2003) 'Quadriceps femoris torque and emg activity in seated versus supine position', *Medicine and Science in Sports and Exercise*, 35(9): 1511–1516.

Osternig, L. R. (1986) 'Isokinetic dynamometry: Implications for muscle testing and rehabilitation', *Exercise and Sport Sciences Reviews*, 14: 45–80.

Pavol, M. J. and Grabiner, M. D. (2000) 'Knee strength variability between individuals across ranges of motion and hip angles', *Medicine and Science in Sports and Exercise*, 32(5): 985–992.

Perrin, D. H. (1993) *Isokinetic Exercise and Assessment*, Champaign, IL: Human Kinetics.

Tsirakos, D., Baltzopoulos, V. and Bartlett, R. (1997) 'Inverse optimization: Functional and physiological considerations related to the force-sharing problem', *Critical Reviews in Biomedical Engineering*, 25(4-5): 371–407.

CHAPTER 7

DATA PROCESSING AND ERROR ESTIMATION

John H. Challis

INTRODUCTION

To paraphrase the English poet Alexander Pope (1688–1744): To err is human; to quantify, divine. Measured values differ from their actual values; they contain errors. Quantification of the errors in any measurement should be made, so that the certainty with which a statement about the results of any analysis is known. Errors can arise during four stages of an analysis process, they are:

- calibration
- acquisition
- data analysis
- data combination

The process of calibration does not eliminate errors but should help keep them to a minimum. Errors owing to calibration occur because a perfect standard for calibration is not feasible; for example, with a motion analysis system the control point positions, used for calibration, are not known to infinite accuracy. Calibration exploits a model to relate a known input to a measurement instrument and, therefore, a change in some aspect of the instrument, to give a desired output. These models are not perfect representations of the system.

During data acquisition errors arise from various sources. These errors can arise because conditions change compared with when calibration was performed; for example, the temperature of the sensors can change. During motion analysis markers attached to the body segments are used to infer underlying bone motion, but the markers typically move relative to the bones (Fuller *et al.*, 1997). For time series data, inappropriately low sample rates can cause errors in sampled data.

Data analysis is the process by which sampled data are further processed to put the data in a usable form. One aspect to consider is that data are normally stored in a digital computer, which means that quantisation errors occur, as do errors owing to finite computer arithmetic. It should be acknowledged that some data analysis procedures can reduce the errors corrupting the sampled data; for example, the low-pass filtering of motion analysis data can have such an effect.

To determine many biomechanical parameters, it is necessary to combine parameters and variables from different sources; in this case, errors arise through the propagation of the errors in the parameters and variables being combined. For example, to compute linear momentum the mass and velocity of an object must be known.

Good experimental practice is to seek to minimise errors at their source; once this has been done, it does not matter what the source of the error is, but it is important to quantify the error. This chapter will outline the terminology used in error analysis, and provide examples of how errors can be both minimised and determined.

DEFINITION OF KEY TERMS

Different terms are used when referring to error analysis, each term has its own specific meaning. To help in reading the subsequent sections, in this section key terms are defined and discussed.

Accuracy

All measurements contain errors; accuracy quantifies the bias in a measure caused by measurement error. Accuracy is quantified as the difference between a true value and an expected/observed value. A measurement made with high accuracy will have little error, or a small bias from the true value. Accuracy is normally specified as the maximum error that can exist in a measurement but, in reality, it is inaccuracy that is being quantified. The term uncertainty is often used interchangeably with accuracy and effectively means the same thing. Accuracy is typically quantified by measuring the deviation between measures and a criterion.

Table 7.1 shows the output from a motion analysis system making 10 repeat measurements on a one-metre long reference moved throughout the field of view of a motion analysis system. Accuracy can be assessed by measuring the bias between the reference length and its measured value. Three evaluation criterion are used, the mean, the absolute mean and the root mean square difference or error. They are calculated as follows:

$$\text{Mean}: \quad \overline{x} = \frac{1}{n} \sum_{i=1}^{n} \Delta x_i \tag{7.1}$$

$$\text{Absolute mean}: \quad \overline{x}_{Abs} = \frac{1}{n} \sum_{i=1}^{n} |\Delta x_i| \tag{7.2}$$

$$\text{Root mean square error}: \text{RMSE} = \sqrt{\frac{\sum_{i=1}^{n} (\Delta x_i)^2}{n}} \tag{7.3}$$

Table 7.1 Ten measures of a reference length measured by a motion analysis system throughout the calibrated volume

Measure	Criterion distance (m)	Measured distance (m)	Difference $[\Delta x_i]$ (cm)
1	1.000	0.9849	−1.51
2	1.000	1.0106	1.06
3	1.000	1.0073	0.73
4	1.000	0.9720	−2.80
5	1.000	0.9964	−0.36
6	1.000	1.0142	1.42
7	1.000	0.9973	−0.27
8	1.000	1.0064	0.64
9	1.000	0.9982	−0.18
10	1.000	0.9962	−0.38
Mean error			−0.17
Absolute mean error			0.93
Root mean square error			1.21

where Δx_i is the difference between a measure and the criterion and n is the number of measurements. The mean value is −0.17 cm but this is not a good measure of accuracy as negative and positive values can cancel one another out, compensating errors. The mean does provide some information, as the tendency is for the system to underestimate lengths. The absolute mean gives a much higher value for the system inaccuracy, 0.93 cm, as does the root mean square difference at 1.21 cm. Adopting the root mean square difference is recommended, as it is the most conservative of the criterion. In this example, accuracy could be expressed as percentage of the field of view of the motion analysis system.

In the above analysis, distances were determined by considering the distance between a pair of markers, so information from this pair of markers had to be combined to compute length. Therefore, the measure of accuracy adopted here does not reflect just the system accuracy as it also includes any error propagated from the combination of data (see below for a description of this problem). Of course, a problem in the assessment of accuracy is finding a suitable criterion with which to compare measured values.

Precision

If a system were measuring something that should remain invariant, deviations in the measured values would indicate a lack of precision. Precision is the difference between an observed and an expected mean value. It is typically

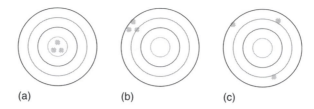

(a)   (b)   (c)

Figure 7.1   Three possible permutations for accuracy and precision, illustrated for shots at the centre of target. (a) High accuracy and high precision. (b) Low accuracy and high precision. (c) Low accuracy and low precision

quantified using the standard deviation of repeat measures of the same quantity:

$$\text{Standard deviation:} \quad \sigma = \left(\frac{1}{n-1} \sum_{i=1}^{n} (x_i - \overline{x})^2 \right)^{\frac{1}{2}} \tag{7.4}$$

Precision and accuracy are sometimes confused, but are distinct quantities. Imagine trying to measure the point of peak pressure beneath the feet during standing using a pedobarograph. If the pedobarograph consists of one sensor only, the system will be very precise, but accuracy in the identification of pressure distributions will be very poor. Figure 7.1 illustrates the three possible permutations for combinations of accuracy and precision, when aiming at a target. Under certain circumstances, precision may be the more important characteristic of a measurement device, for example if looking at changes in joint angles because of some intervention.

Resolution

For any measurement instrument there is a limit on the measured quantity, which produces a change in the output of the instrument. Therefore, resolution reflects the 'fineness' with which a measurement can be made. Often resolution is expressed as a value or as a percentage of the instrument's full measuring range. If a measuring tape is used to determine segment perimeter length then the resolution of the tape is indicated by the smallest sub-division on the tape. For example, if the tape is marked in 2 mm increments it may be reasonable to resolve measures to 1 mm. With electronic measurement instruments, reporting measures to many decimal places does not necessarily indicate high resolution, as a large component of these values may reflect system noise.

Noise

Errors corrupting sampled data are referred to as noise. Noise is the unwanted part of sampled data; it masks the true value in which the experimenter is interested. Noise should be minimised in sampled data before further processing of the signal. The noise can be either systematic or random.

Systematic noise

Systematic noise is a signal superimposed over the true signal, which varies systematically and is correlated in some way with the measurement process, or the thing being measured. For example, the use of weights to calibrate a force plate could cause systematic error if their weight was one per cent less than that assumed during calibration. Many sources of systematic noise can often be modelled during the calibration process and removed from the sampled signal.

Random noise

Random noise is a signal superimposed over the true signal, which is typically described as being 'white'. White noise is random in the sense that the noise signal is stationary, has a mean value of zero and a flat power spectrum.

Propagated error

To perform biomechanical analyses, different mechanical parameters have to be combined, so different sources of error impinge on the derived mechanical variable. Propagated error is the error that occurs in one operation and spreads into other operations. The section in this chapter on Combination of Variables and Parameters demonstrates the mathematical principles behind error propagation. In the following sections, it is the intention to review the ways in which uncertainties can be assessed and minimised for the main data collection and processing techniques used in biomechanics.

SAMPLING TIME SERIES DATA

In many applications data is collected at multiple instants. The interval between samples may be months, as when measuring growth curves, or milliseconds if measuring centre of pressure motion during quiet stance. There are some basic principles that govern the collection of time series data; these will be discussed in this section.

The sampling theorem gained widespread acceptance through the work of Claude Shannon; it states that a signal should be sampled at a rate that is greater than twice the highest frequency component in the signal. This seems a simple concept but, before data collection, how does the experimenter know the highest frequency component of the signal? Previously published studies and pilot studies will provide useful guidelines, but if a participant exhibits strange behaviour then this option may not be appropriate. A general guideline is to sample at a rate ten times greater than the anticipated highest frequency in the signal. Selecting such a high sample rate provides a safeguard if the analysed movement contains higher frequency components than normally expected. There are some additional advantages to a higher sample rate, which are outlined at the end of this section.

If the sampling theorem is not followed, the sampled signal will be aliased, which means that any frequency components higher than the Nyquist frequency (half of the sampling rate) will be folded back into the sampled frequency domain. Therefore, it is essential for the accurate analysis of time series data that the signal be sampled at a sufficiently high sample rate, although it is not normal to know a priori the frequency content of a signal. For example, signal 1 has a maximum frequency content of 1 Hz and is sampled at 8 Hz, and signal 2 has a maximum frequency content of 7 Hz and is also sampled at 8 Hz. Figure 7.2 shows that signal 1 is adequately sampled, but signal 2 is not.

When sampling any signal the experimenter is guided by Shannon's sampling theorem, which in essence states that any band-limited signal can be unambiguously reconstructed when that signal is sampled at a rate greater than twice the band-limit of the signal. Slepain, 1976, has shown that, theoretically, no signal is band-limited but, for practical implementation, the assumption is

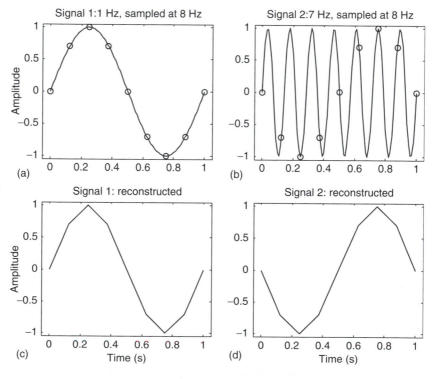

Figure 7.2 Illustration of the influence of sample rate on reconstructed signal, where 'o' indicates a sampled data point

made that the signal is band-limited. Often overlooked in Shannon's work is the interpolation formula presented, which allows the sampled signal to represent the original analogue (Shannon, 1948). The use of a sample rate of only just greater than twice the band-limit of the signal allows accurate representation of the signal in the frequency domain but not in the time domain. Figure 7.3 shows a signal with frequency components up to 3 Hz, which has been sampled at two different rates, 10 and 100 Hz. The 10 Hz sampled signal while representing the frequency components of the sampled signal provides poor temporal resolution. For example, estimates of the minimum and maximum values of the signal in the 10 Hz sampled version of the signal produces an error of just under six per cent. The temporal resolution of the signal can be increased by interpolating the data; in Figure 7.3 the datasets have been interpolated using a cubic spline; now the signals at both sample rates are equivalent. Therefore, under certain conditions further processing is warranted to produce from the sampled data a good representation of the signal in the time domain.

For certain applications sample duration can be as important as sample rate. The lowest frequency that can be determined from collected data depends

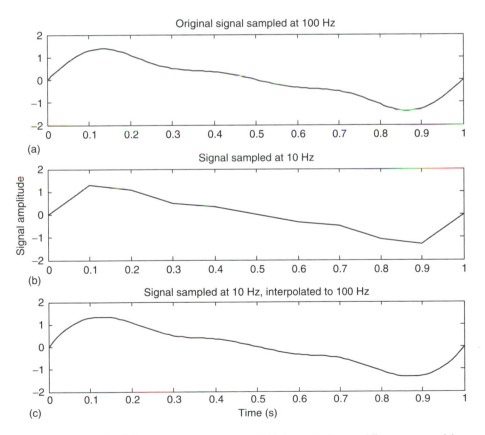

Figure 7.3 A signal with frequency components up to 3 Hz is sampled at two different rates, and then interpolated to a greater temporal density

on the duration of the sample. If for a particular task the low frequency components of the signal are important then sample duration should be appropriately selected.

In most analyses it is assumed that random noise contaminating the data is white. One of the assumptions for white noise is that it contains all frequencies. Under this assumption some noise will always be aliased, as there is noise that exists beyond the Nyquist rate; this noise will be folded back in to the sampled domain. The appropriate sampling of a signal should also focus on adequate sampling of the noise. If the noise is small compared with the signal, then a low sample rate may be appropriate as noise aliasing may not be a problem. If the noise is large compared with the signal, then a high sample rate may be appropriate.

The following recommendations are made:

- Data should be sampled at a sufficiently high sampling frequency to avoid signal aliasing.
- Signals should be sampled at a rate ten times greater than the anticipated highest frequency in the signal, as this provides a safety margin, should the frequency content of the movement be atypical.
- After appropriate sampling of data, signal interpolation to provide greater temporal resolution should be considered.
- If low frequencies are of interest sample duration should be appropriately selected.

IMAGE-BASED MOTION ANALYSIS AND RECONSTRUCTION ACCURACY

A common method used in biomechanics is to collect motion information from analysis of the images of the task. These images can be registered digitally or on to film or video. There are various methods by which calibration and reconstruction can be performed; these include the direct linear transformation (Abdel-Aziz and Karara, 1971), simultaneous multi-frame analytical calibration (Woltring, 1980), the non-linear transformation technique (Dapena *et al.*, 1982) and wand calibration (Borghese *et al.*, 2001). The worthwhile application of any of these techniques depends on the resulting accuracy and precision. Accuracy can be assessed by looking at the difference between the true and measured locations of points, precision as the repeatability with which a measure can be made. Accuracy will depend on both the digitising procedure and the reconstruction technique, while precision will be more dependent on the digitising.

Accuracy has commonly been reported for image-based motion analysis as the difference between the true location of the control points and their predicted values. Challis and Kerwin, 1992, have shown that using the same control points for calibration and accuracy assessment overestimates accuracy; therefore, a second independent set of control points is essential if control points are used for accuracy assessment. There are alternatives to using control points to assess accuracy, for example a rod of known length can be moved throughout the calibrated space and the difference between its true length and predicted length compared. Wood and Marshall, 1986, and Challis, 1995a, have shown how the commonly used direct linear transformation technique produces less accurate predictions of the locations of points outside of the volume encompassed by the control points compared with those inside this volume. These studies highlight the need to assess the accuracy of reconstruction throughout the space in which the activity takes place even if this is greater than the space encompassed by the control points.

It should not be assumed that, because similar or the same equipment is being used as in other studies, the reconstruction accuracy is the same. Many factors influence reconstruction accuracy and a small change in one may change the accuracy of reconstruction. For example, Abdel-Aziz, 1974, showed how the angle between the intersections of the optical axes of the cameras causes different reconstruction accuracy.

Landmarks are either naturally occurring, such as a bony protuberance, or a marker of some kind is placed on the skin surface to specify the position and orientation of the segments with which they are associated. These landmarks or markers may not always be visible from all camera views, in which case their location has to estimated. Skin movement can affect the ability of a marker to stay over the bony landmark it is intended to represent (Fuller *et al.*, 1997). Assessment of inter-marker distance, for markers on the same segment, will reflect system accuracy, precision and marker movement. Such an assessment provides a simple means of assessing the marker motion.

When digitising manually, there are two types of precision: that of a single operator and that between operators. The main operator should digitise some sequences at least twice to get an estimate of precision, evaluated using the root mean square difference between the two measures. If more time is available, the operator should perform multiple digitisations of the same sequence, in which case precision can be estimated by computing the standard deviation. It could be that the operator is particularly imprecise, or is introducing a systematic error into the measurement process, for example by consistently digitising the wrong body landmark. Therefore, it is also recommended that a second operator digitise at least one sequence; this should quickly identify any systematic errors introduced by one of the digitisers, and it also gives a measure of inter-operator precision. Such an assessment analyses objectivity, if a low level of precision is evident between operators, then the assessment requires a high degree of subjective assessment to evaluate body landmark positions. Once precision has been quantified, the effect of this precision on variables computed from the position data should be evaluated.

Problems of marker location and identification can be particularly acute with automated image-based motion analysis systems for which, if a marker is obscured from a camera view, reconstruction may not be possible; after this loss, the subsequent identification of markers may be problematic. Under these conditions either the operator is asked to make an estimate or the software attempts to make an 'educated guess' as to where the marker is. These influences should be assessed using the protocols just described. It should also be appreciated that with multiple camera systems a marker's position may be reconstructed from a variable number of cameras throughout an activity, resulting in changes in marker position accuracy.

The following recommendations are made:

- Reconstruction accuracy should be assessed using the root mean square difference between true control point locations and their estimated locations.
- The control points used for accuracy assessment should be independent of those used for calibration.
- If control points are not available a rod of known length with markers on either end can be used for accuracy assessment, as long as it is moved throughout the calibrated volume.
- Analysing movements that occur outside of the calibrated volume should be avoided.

BODY SEGMENT INERTIAL PARAMETERS

For many biomechanical analyses it is often necessary to know the inertial parameters of the body segments involved, which, for biomechanical assessment, normally include the mass, moments of inertia and location of the centre of mass of each segment. Unfortunately, there are no ready measures of accuracy for individual segmental parameters. What can be assessed is the relative influence of different inertial parameter sets on other variables or parameters computed using the inertial parameters. For example Challis, 1996, made three estimates of the moments of inertia of the segments of the lower limb; the resultant joint moments were then estimated at the ankle, knee and hip using each of the inertial parameter estimates. The percentage root mean square differences between the various estimates of the resultant joint moments were then assessed. For the two activities examined, maximum vertical jumping and walking, there was little difference between resultant joint moments with the percentage root mean square differences all less than two per cent irrespective of which moment of inertia values were used. Such an approach has been extended by Challis and Kerwin, 1996, to include all inertial parameters. This is not a direct assessment of accuracy but it facilitates evaluation of the influence of possible inaccuracies in inertial parameters. Given such an assessment it should be possible to conclude that the inertial parameters have been computed with sufficient accuracy for the analysis to be undertaken, if the influences of different inertial parameter estimates are within tolerable ranges.

Mungiole and Martin, 1990, compared the inertial parameters estimated using different techniques with the results obtained from magnetic resonance imaging of the lower limbs of 12 males. These results are reassuring in that they show that different techniques all give very similar estimates of body segment inertial parameters. It could be decided to take one set and then perturbate that set by amounts that reflect the potential accuracy of that inertial parameter estimation procedure, rather than to take the measurements required to make different estimates of the segment inertial parameters. In this case, an estimate of the accuracy of the inertial parameters is required; here the data of Mungiole and Martin, 1990, could be used for the lower limb. Yeadon and Morlock, 1989, evaluated the error in estimating human body segment moments of inertia using both linear and non-linear equations, providing another source of data on which perturbations could be performed.

With certain methods for determining body segment inertial parameters, some measures of accuracy are possible. For example, if the method predicts the mass of the segments, these can be summed for all segments to give an estimate of whole body mass, which can be compared with actual body mass. Unfortunately only one parameter is being assessed and compensating errors may mask genuine accuracy. When modelling the body as a series of geometric solids it is possible to compare model predicted segment volume with actual volume (e.g. Hatze, 1980); volume is not normally required for biomechanical analyses, although it does have a bearing on the accuracy of estimated masses.

The following recommendation is made:

- As there are no ready measures of accuracy for the inertial parameters of body segments, sensitivity analysis of these parameters should be performed.

LOW-PASS FILTERING AND COMPUTATION OF DERIVATIVES

For many biomechanical analyses it is necessary to reduce the white noise that contaminates the sampled data by low-pass filtering. For example, with image-based motion analysis data it is assumed that the movement signal occupies the low frequencies and that the noise is present across all frequencies; to reduce the influence of noise the data are low-pass filtered. As white noise exists across the frequency spectrum some noise will still remain in the signal. There are various methods used in biomechanics for low-pass filtering data, which can be placed into three broad categories:

- digital filters, such as the Butterworth filter (Winter *et al.*, 1974)
- splines; for example, generalised cross-validated quintic spline (e.g. Woltring, 1986)
- frequency domain techniques, such as the truncated Fourier Series (e.g. Hatze, 1981).

To an extent all of these approaches are equivalent (Craven and Wahba, 1979). After low-pass filtering the data appears smoother; thus, low-pass filtering is sometimes referred to as smoothing.

In some applications it is also necessary to compute signal derivatives. In the frequency domain signal differentiation is equivalent to signal amplification, with increasing amplification with increasing frequency. A simple example illustrates the influence of data differentiation on signal components. Assume that the true signal is a simple sine wave with an amplitude of 1; this will be corrupted by noise across the spectrum but this example will focus on only one noise component with an amplitude of 0.001. The signal to noise ratio can be computed for the zero, first and second order derivatives:

Displacement: $x(t) = \sin t$;   Noise $(t) = 0.001\sin 50t$;   Signal to noise ratio: 1:0.001.
Velocity: $v(t) = \cos t$;   Noise $(t) = 0.05\cos 50t$;   Signal to noise ratio: 1:0.05.
Acceleration: $a(t) = -\sin t$;   Noise $(t) = -2.5\sin 50t$;   Signal to noise ratio: 1:2.5.

This example illustrates how important it is to low-pass filter data before data differentiation to reduce the high frequency noise components of the sampled signal.

The question arises of how to select the amount of filtering or smoothing. If the properties of the signal and noise were known then the amount of the filtering could easily be selected, but this is not the case. If too low a cut-off is selected, the resulting signal will be incorrect as data from the original signal will have been discarded; if, on the other hand, the cut-off is too high then too much noise will remain in the signal.

To specify the amount of filtering some researchers use previously published values, but this approach makes many assumptions about the similarity of experimental set-up and participant performance across studies. It also assumes that the original researchers made an appropriate selection. A range of procedures is available to determine automatically the amount of filtering. These approaches try to use information present in the sampled data to determine the amount of filtering; typically they assume that the noise is white. Hatze, 1981, based on the work of Anderssen and Bloomfield, 1974, presented an automatic procedure for using truncated Fourier series to low-pass filter and differentiate noisy data. Craven and Wahba (1979) presented a generalised cross-validation procedure for identifying optimal smoothing. This method fits a function to the data and determines the degree of fit, which minimises the root mean square fit to the data if each point in the data is systematically removed, and the fit is assessed by sequentially estimating these points. The generalised cross-validated quintic spline is most appropriate for the order of derivatives that are typically required in biomechanics (Woltring et al., 1985). To estimate the appropriate cut-off for a Butterworth filter, Challis, 1999, exploited the properties of the autocorrelation of white noise.

To illustrate some of the differences between these techniques, the performances of a Butterworth filter with the cut-off frequency selected using an autocorrelation procedure (Challis, 1999) and a quintic spline with the degree of smoothing selected using a generalised cross-validation procedure (Woltring, 1986) were evaluated. Dowling, 1985, presented data for which he simultaneously collected accelerometer data and motion-analysis displacement data. Figure 7.4 presents the estimates for the two techniques of the accelerometer data, along with the actual acceleration data. Notice that the autocorrelation procedure underestimates the peak acceleration values (Figure 7.4c), but performs better than the generalised cross-validated quintic spline around the region of limited acceleration (Figure 7.4d).

These automatic procedures are all, to some extent, 'black-box' techniques, which should be used with caution. Their advantage is that they remove

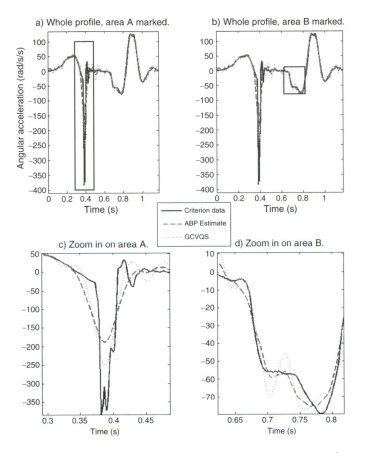

Figure 7.4 The performance of two filtering and differentiating techniques, autocorrelation procedure (ABP) and generalised cross-validated quintic spline (GCVQS), for estimating acceleration data from noisy displacement data using criterion acceleration data of Dowling, 1985

some subjectivity in assessing the degree of filtering, and, thereby, can provide consistency between studies.

Consider a gymnast rotating around a high bar; if the analysis focuses on wrist and knee motion, the linear motion of the wrist will be much smaller than that of the knee. The noise arising from a motion analysis system will be equivalent for the wrist and the knee, yet the range of motion is different so they have different signal-to-noise ratios. Therefore, for this example it does not make sense to select the same smoothing for both landmarks. The same is true for many activities: different landmarks have different signal-to-noise ratios, so require different amounts of filtering.

Lanshammar, 1982, presented a series of formulae that provides an estimate of the noise that can be expected to remain in a noisy signal after smoothing and or differentiation. The basic formula is:

$$\sigma_k^2 \geq \frac{\sigma^2 \tau \omega_b^{2k+1}}{\pi (2k+1)} \tag{7.5}$$

where σ_k^2 is the minimum variance of the noise affecting the kth derivative, after processing, σ^2 is the variance of the additive white noise, τ is the sample interval, ω_b is the bandwidth of the signal in radians per second ($\omega_b = 2\pi f_b$), and f_b is the sample bandwidth in Hz. Equation 7.5 highlights several important points:

- Appropriate low-pass filtering of the data will reduce noise.
- Derivatives will always be of less precision than the original data.
- To increase data precision you have to decrease the variance of the additive white noise (σ^2) or decrease the sample interval (τ); the latter effectively means increasing the sampling rate.
- Signal bandwidth is the final variable in equation 7.5, but is determined by the activity so cannot be adjusted by the experimenter.

There are three major assumptions associated with the formula of Lanshammar, 1982, which mean that it gives only minimum estimates. The assumptions are:

1   The signal is band-limited; however, mathematically no signal is band-limited (Slepian, 1976). Effectively frequencies above the Nyquist frequency are ignored.
2   The noise contaminating the signal is white; however, it is unrealistic that the noise corrupting a signal would be perfectly white.
3   The frequency response of the filter or differentiator is ideal. An ideal low-pass filter passes a signal unattenuated up to the specified filter cut-off, after which the entire remaining signal is removed irrespective of whether it is noise or true signal. An ideal differentiator must suitably amplify a signal up to the cut-off frequency after which no signal is allowed to pass. Such filters and differentiators are not practically realisable.

It is evident from equation 7.5 that a figure of merit for comparing different analysis systems is the product $\sigma\sqrt{\tau}$. Using this figure it is possible to compare the relative balance between a system that produces little noise at a low sample rate with one that produces noisier data but at a higher sample rate.

To use this formula the variance of the additive white noise is required. Even if derivatives are not going to be calculated and the raw data are used, the noise should still be estimated. If the noise contaminating a signal is white, this means the noise is not correlated between samples and has a mean value of zero. On summing repeat measures the true underlying signal is additive, and the noise tends to its mean value. Therefore, taking the mean of repeat samples, the signal to noise ratio is improved. If n repeat measures are taken, the true signal size is increased by a factor n, the variance of the noise is increased by the same factor, while the standard deviation of the noise is increased by a factor equal to the square root of n. On taking the mean, the ratio of the signal amplitude to the noise standard deviation is increased by the square root of n.

Winter *et al.*, 1974, estimated noise levels by quantifying the variation in the location of a marker on the foot when the foot was stationary during the stance phase of gait. Such an analysis does not provide information about the noise affecting all of the sampled data and has limited application in other activities. When quantifying the accuracy of derivative information if whole body motion has been analysed, the ground reaction forces can be estimated during ground contact and then compared with force plate records, or the accelerations can be compared to gravitational acceleration during free flight. Such an analysis is not a direct way of assessing signal quality as body segment inertial parameters are also required.

The following recommendations are made:

- Low-pass filtering of data is recommended, and is imperative if derivatives are to be computed.
- Different landmarks on the body will typically require different amounts of filtering.
- Selection of the amount of filtering should be prudently done, with an automated procedure recommended.
- Estimation of the noise that can be expected to remain in a noisy signal after filtering and differentiation can be performed using the formula of Lanshammar, 1982.
- To compare motion analysis systems with different sample rates and noise levels, the following figure of merit should be used: $\sigma\sqrt{\tau}$.

SEGMENT ORIENTATION AND JOINT ANGLES

When defining angles in either two or three dimensions, the rotations defined relate the transformation of one reference frame on to another. For example segment orientation may be defined by relating an inertial reference frame to a reference frame defined for the segment. The transformation of coordinates measured in the segment reference frame to the inertial reference frame can be represented by:

$$y_i = [R]x_i + v \tag{7.6}$$

where y_i is the position of point i on the segment measured in the inertial reference frame, $[R]$ is the attitude matrix, x_i is the position of point i on the segment measured in the segment reference frame, and v is the position of the origin of segment reference frame in the inertial reference frame. Matrix $[R]$ is a proper orthonormal matrix, which, therefore, has the following properties:

$$[R]^T[R] = [R][R]^T = [R]^{-1}[R] = [I] \tag{7.7}$$
$$det([R]) = +1 \tag{7.8}$$

where $[I]$ is the identity matrix, and $det([R])$ denotes the determinant of matrix $[R]$.

Once determined, angles can be extracted from the matrix $[R]$; for a two-dimensional analysis, one angle and, for a three-dimensional analysis, three angles. There are several procedures for determining this matrix; a comparison of various approaches suggests the least-squares approach currently produces the most accurate results (Challis, 1995b). In a least-squares sense the task of determining $[R]$ and v is equivalent to minimising

$$\frac{1}{n} \sum_{i=1}^{n} ([R]x_i + v - y_i)^T ([R]x_i + v - y_i) \tag{7.9}$$

where n is the number of common landmarks measured in both reference frames ($n \geq 2$ for two-dimensional analyses, $n \geq 3$ for three-dimensional analyses).

The computation techniques for minimising equation 7.9 include those presented by Veldpaus *et al.*, 1988, and Challis, 1995b; 2001a, for two-dimensional analysis. Both the number of markers on a segment and their distribution influence the accuracy with which equation 7.9 is solved and, therefore, the resulting angles extracted from $[R]$ (Challis, 1995c).

Given the locations of landmarks on the body of interest, it is then common practice to determine the orientations of the body segments and the relative orientation of adjacent segments (joint angles). In two dimensions these segment orientations are normally computed by defining landmarks at the distal and proximal ends of the segment, the angle between a line joining these marks and the horizontal is then computed. It is possible to compute the precision with which these angles are measured using the following formula:

$$\sigma_\phi^2 = \frac{2 \cdot \sigma^2}{l^2} \tag{7.10}$$

where σ_ϕ^2 is the error variance of the angle, σ^2 is the error variance of the noise affecting the co-ordinates and l^2 is the distance between markers or body landmarks. The error variance of the noise affecting the co-ordinates can be estimated using the methods described in the previous section. The equation shows that to increase the accuracy of the angle computation the noise affecting the co-ordinates should be minimised, and that the distance between the markers should be maximised. In the analysis of human movement there is a limit to the distance markers can be separated on a segment and marker locations must also be selected considering other factors, such as minimising underlying skin movement, making sure the markers are visible to cameras and marking anatomically meaningful sites. These same principles apply to the determination of angles in three dimensions (Challis, 1995a). The error variance of the angle could also be arrived at by computing the angle several times from repeat measurements and using this to establish the variance of the estimation.

If an angle is described in three dimensions then, in biomechanics, these angles are normally defined as an ordered set of three rotations about a specified set of axes; in effect, each angle is associated with a rotation about a given axis4. The error variances in three dimensions are influenced in a similar way to angles in two dimensions (Woltring, 1994). The errors in the three angles are highly correlated and cannot be considered independent when analysing signal noise. For the Cardanic angle convention the influence of noise becomes greater when the middle angle approaches $\pm(2n+1)\pi/2$, where n is any integer. At these angles the other two (terminal) angles are undefined; the angle system has a singularity.

The other commonly used system for defining angles is the Eulerian system, with the singularity for this angle system occurring when the middle angle approaches $\pm n\pi$. Angle conventions and axes orientations should be selected not only to avoid singularities but also to keep the angles from approaching these singularities. Woltring, 1994, has presented an angle set which avoids the singularities inherent in Eulerian or Cardanic angles and whose covariances are better, the so-called helical angles; the disadvantage is that this angle definition lacks any physical significance. A similar critique can be levelled at other methods for parameterising the attitude matrix, which extract four parameters from the matrix, such as Euler parameters and quaternions.

It should be noted that the error analyses presented in this section assumes that the error affecting the co-ordinates used to compute the angles is isotropic. This is not always the case as some analysis systems have different resolutions in different directions. For example, in three-dimensional analysis using video cameras the depth axis – that perpendicular to a line between the principal points of a two-camera system – is often measured with lower accuracy than the other two axes. Under conditions of anisotropic noise there may be increased error effects, although in most biomechanical applications noise is normally only mildly anisotropic.

Sometimes helical or screw axes are used to quantify joint motions. Although beyond the scope of this chapter, Woltring et al., 1985, presented formulae for the estimation of the error variance associated with estimating the helical axis parameters. If these variables are to be used to examine joint motion, the reader is directed to this work.

The following recommendations are made:

*   As many markers as feasible should be used to define a segment.
*   The markers should be distributed as far apart as possible, while avoiding areas where skin motion may be large.
*   In three-dimensions the angle definition system should be selected so that singularities, or approaching these singularities, are avoided for the movement to be analysed.

FORCE PLATES

Force plates are normally used to measure the ground reaction forces and the centre of pressure. Hall et al., 1996, presented a procedure for the static calibration of force plates, which allows calibration or confirmation of calibration for the three force and moment directions with checks for cross-talk between axes. The method was used to evaluate a Kistler 9261A force plate and the results of this evaluation comfortingly confirmed the factory calibrations. Bobbert and Schamhardt, 1990, by point loading, examined the accuracy of the centre of pressure estimates of a force plate. They were able to show that there were large errors in the centre of pressure estimates using the plate particularly toward the edges; they also presented equations to correct for these errors. Their analysis was for a larger model of force plate; the errors may not be so large for smaller plates. Particularly in cases where the force plate is not installed in line with manufacturer's specifications these checks should be mandatory.

Another less-considered problem with the force plate is the natural frequency of the plate. Any object when struck will vibrate, the frequency of the vibration is called the natural frequency. Many objects, particularly if they are composed of number different materials, have several frequencies at which they vibrate. It is normal to report a force plate's lowest natural frequency. The anticipation is that the frequency of the movement being analysed is lower than the natural frequency of the force plate, in which case the two can easily be separated; this appears to be the case for commercially available plates mounted according to manufacturer's specifications. If the amplitude of the natural frequencies is low then these can be ignored, if this is not the case they should be filtered and removed from the sampled data, ideally before the data are converted from an analogue to a digital form. Manufacturers reported natural frequencies only apply if the force plate is mounted according to manufacturer's specifications (Kerwin and Chapman, 1988); if this is not the case, the natural frequency of the plate should be examined; then either the plate mounting should be modified or the analogue signal appropriately high-pass filtered.

It is not the intention of this chapter to discuss the precision or accuracy with which human movement can be analysed if the participant is considered, but it should be mentioned that in biomechanics there have been several studies looking at the repeatability of force plate measures. These studies include the influence of targeting and not targeting the force plate (walking – Grabiner *et al.*, 1995; running – Challis, 2001b), and how many times a participant should run over the plate to get a representative ground reaction force pattern (e.g. Bates *et al.*, 1983). In designing a study using the force plate the experimenter is advised to bear these factors in mind.

The analogue force data are converted into digital form for storage and analysis on a computer. The digitised values are each a single packet of information (word), represented in binary form; for example 10110 (binary) = 22 (decimal). Each word contains a certain amount of information (bits), which varies with word length; for example, 10110 (binary) contains 5 bits of information. The more bits of information, the higher is the resolution of the system. For example, if the input signal is 0 to 10 volts, and the analogue to digital converter has a resolution of 10 bits, then a single count would represent,

$$\frac{10}{2^{10}} = \frac{10}{1024} = 0.0098 \, \text{volts} \approx 0.01 \, \text{volts} \tag{7.11}$$

It is feasible to resolve to half a count, therefore, the quantising error is 0.005 V. Depending on the signal to be analysed and the measuring equipment, quantising error may be very significant, as in Figure 7.5.

To determine resultant joint moments, often information from a force plate and a motion analysis system are combined. Poor alignment between the force plate and motion analysis system reference frames can cause large errors in the computed moments (McCaw and Devita, 1995). Calibration procedures and calibration checking routines should be used to ensure these two references frames are appropriately aligned (e.g. Rabuffetti *et al.*, 2003).

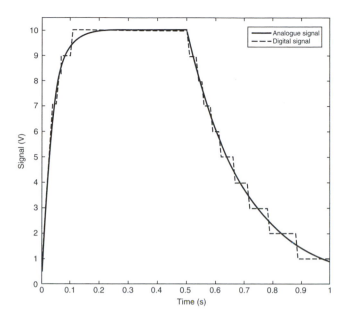

Figure 7.5   Example of quantisation error, where the resolution only permits resolution to 1 volt

The following recommendations are made:

- Confirm factory calibration of the force plate.
- If a force plate cannot be mounted to manufacturer's specifications, then the natural frequency of the plate should be determined.
- An analogue filter should be considered for removing force components generated by the natural frequency of the force plate.
- The resolution of the analogue-to-digital converter should be matched to the required accuracy of the force measures.
- When the force plate is used in combination with a motion analysis system, it should be confirmed that the force plate and motion analysis system reference frames are aligned.

COMBINATION OF VARIABLES AND PARAMETERS

For any parameters or state variables, an uncertainty is associated with their estimation; these uncertainties will propagate in any value determined from their combination. The uncertainty in any value determined from a combination of parameters or state variables can be expressed mathematically (Barford, 1985). If the required state variable is P, which is a function of n state variables or parameters then:

$$P = f(X_1, X_2, \ldots, X_n) \tag{7.12}$$

$$(\delta P)^2 = \sum_{i=1}^{n} \left[\frac{\partial P}{\partial X_i} \delta X_i \right]^2 \tag{7.13}$$

where X_i is a state variable, δP is the uncertainty in the variable P, $\dfrac{\partial P}{\partial X_i}$ is the partial derivative of function P with respect to X_i, and δX_i is the uncertainty in variable X_i. Equation 7.13 shows how errors in the variables, or parameters required to compute another parameter or variable, propagate to produce an error in the computed value. For example if the function is the addition or subtraction of two variables then:

$$P = f(x, y) = x \pm y \tag{7.14}$$

$$\frac{\partial P}{\partial x} = \frac{\partial P}{\partial y} = 1 \tag{7.15}$$

$$\delta P^2 = \left(\frac{\partial P}{\partial x}\delta x\right)^2 + \left(\frac{\partial P}{\partial y}\delta y\right)^2 = \delta x^2 + \delta y^2 \tag{7.16}$$

For the multiplication of two variables:

$$P = f(x, y) = xy \tag{7.17}$$

$$(\delta P)^2 = (y\delta x)^2 + (x\delta y)^2 \tag{7.18}$$

Note that when combining two variables, it is not a simple case of adding or taking the mean of the errors in two variables to compute the error in the derived variable. If the variable P is dependent on many other variables, then equation 7.14 becomes quite unwieldy. Performing such an analysis assumes that the uncertainties in the variables are random and uncorrelated. Equations 7.16 and 7.18 can easily be used for simple biomechanical analyses; for more complex biomechanical analyses the resulting system of equations derived from equation 7.13 can become unwieldy.

Another way to assess the influence of these uncertainties, which does not require the same assumptions and is a potentially simpler one, is to perform a sensitivity analysis, where the parameters and state variables are changed, or perturbated, by amounts relating to the estimated uncertainty or error with which they were measured. The change in the required state variable because of this perturbation is then quantified. The main problem associated with assessing uncertainty in this way is how to allow for all the possible combinations of potential errors. Figure 7.6 shows the rectangular parallelepiped that contains all possible combinations of the errors if, for example, the calculation of a key variable requires the combination of three variables (x, y and z). The figure illustrates that you theoretically have infinite possible combinations of the errors. To some extent this problem can be viewed as a programming problem, as an appropriately written computer program can easily investigate a reasonable sub-set of the options. Writing software for this purpose can be problematic and many commercial software packages are not written with such flexibility. A commonly used compromise is to run calculations for nine of the possible error options, one with the original data set with no noise (the origin in the figure), and each of the corners of the rectangular parallelepiped. The assumption here is that the larger the error the larger its resulting effect on any variable derived from using it; therefore, considering the combinations using the maximum errors examines

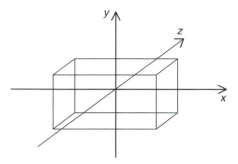

Figure 7.6 Graph showing the rectangular parallelepiped which encompasses all possible error combinations in variables x, y and z

the maximum error condition for the derived variable. In most cases, this is generally true although, if time permits, examining more than nine of the possible options is recommended.

If the uncertainty is quantified using either of the methods just discussed, then the problem of how to estimate the error in the variables and parameters still remains. The solution to this problem is to use a direct procedure where possible, for example procedures similar to those outlined earlier in this chapter, or to take an appropriate figure from the literature. Selection of values from the literature should be done prudently by matching the selected published study to yours as closely as possible.

The following recommendations are made:

*   Error propagation formulae can be used to quantify the error when two or more unrelated measures are combined.
*   Otherwise a sensitivity analysis should be used to estimate errors.

CONCLUSIONS

There are many measurement procedures used in biomechanics, which are too numerous to cover in detail here. The preceding should have provided sufficient information to enable measurement accuracy to be assessed for other devices or procedures. Software for processing data, in the ways described in this chapter, is available from several sources. Basic signal processing software is available in MATLAB (http://www.mathworks.com/), and the freely available GNU Octave (http://www.octave.org/). More biomechanics specific code can be downloaded from the web site of the International Society of Biomechanics (http://www.isbweb.org/).

The following broad recommendations are made:

*   With any measurement procedure, it is important to follow the basic experimental protocols, which means that the equipment must be accurately calibrated.

- Accuracy of calibration should be assessed using an independent measurement that assesses the accuracy throughout the range of required measurements.
- For time series data, the sampling rate should be selected to avoid signal aliasing.
- Errors should be estimated and reported for all measurements.
- If the measurements are combined to derive further variables or parameters it is essential that the effect of combining errors from different sources is quantified and reported.

It is not possible to set acceptable magnitudes of uncertainty, as these will vary from study to study. The purpose of the study dictates what the acceptable uncertainty is; a pedantic search for increased accuracy with a particular measuring device may be redundant for the purpose of one study and yet be essential for another. Some of the factors that affect uncertainties cannot be known a priori, for example, the bandwidth of the sampled signal. When the measurement uncertainty cannot be sufficiently well estimated before data collection, a strict adherence to good experimental protocols followed by an error analysis is the experimenter's only recourse. Although the analysis of errors can be tiresome, it does give one the satisfaction of knowing what confidence can be placed on the results and any conclusions drawn from them.

REFERENCES

Abdel-Aziz, Y.I. (1974) 'Expected accuracy of convergent photos', *Photogrammetric Engineering*, 40: 1341–1346.

Abdel-Aziz, Y.I. and Karara, H.M. (1971) 'Direct linear transformation from comparator co-ordinates into object space co-ordinates in close range photogrammetry', in *American Society of Photogrammetry Symposium on Close Range Photogrammetry*, Falls Church, VA: American Society of Photogrammetry.

Anderssen, R.S. and Bloomfield, P. (1974) 'Numerical differentiation procedures for non-exact data', *Numerische Mathematik*, 22: 157–182.

Barford, N.C. (1985) *Experimental Measurements: Precision, Error and Truth*, New York: John Wiley.

Bates, B.T.L., Osternig, L.R., Sawhill, J.A. and James, S.L. (1983) 'An assessment of subject variability, subject–shoe interaction, and the evaluation of running shoes using ground reaction force data', *Journal of Biomechanics*, 16: 181–191.

Bobbert, M.F. and Schamhardt, H.C. (1990) 'Accuracy of determining the point of force application with piezoelectric force plates', *Journal of Biomechanics*, 23: 705–710.

Borghese, N.A., Cerveri, P. and Rigiroli, P. (2001) 'A fast method for calibrating video-based motion analysers using only a rigid bar', *Medical and Biological Engineering and Computing*, 39: 76–81.

Challis, J.H. (1995a) 'A multiphase calibration procedure for the Direct Linear Transformation', *Journal of Applied Biomechanics*, 11: 351–358.

Challis, J.H. (1995b) 'An examination of procedures for determining body segment attitude and position from noisy biomechanical data', *Medical Engineering and Physics*, 17: 83–90.

Challis, J.H. (1995c) 'A procedure for determining rigid body transformation parameters', *Journal of Biomechanics*, 28: 733–737.

Challis, J.H. (1996) 'The evaluation of the accuracy of human limb moment of inertias and their influence on resultant joint moments', *Journal of Applied Biomechanics*, 12: 515–529.

Challis, J.H. (1999) 'A procedure for the automatic determination of filter cutoff frequency of the processing of biomechanical data', *Journal of Applied Biomechanics*, 15: 303–317.

Challis, J.H. (2001a) 'Estimation of the finite center of rotation in planar movements', *Medical Engineering and Physics*, 23: 227–233.

Challis, J.H. (2001b) 'The variability in running gait caused by force plate targeting', *Journal of Applied Biomechanics*, 17: 77–83.

Challis, J.H. and Kerwin, D.G. (1992) 'Accuracy assessment and control point configuration when using the DLT for cine-photogrammetry', *Journal of Biomechanics*, 25: 1053–1058.

Challis, J.H. and Kerwin, D.G. (1996) 'Quantification of the uncertainties in resultant joint moments computed in a dynamic activity', *Journal of Sports Sciences*, 14: 219–231.

Craven, P. and Wahba, G. (1979) 'Smoothing noisy data with spline functions: Estimating the correct degree of smoothing by the method of generalised cross-validation', *Numerische Mathematik*, 31: 377–403.

Dapena, J., Harman, E.A. and Miller, J.A. (1982) 'Three-dimensional cinematography with control object of unknown shape', *Journal of Biomechanics*, 15: 11–19.

Dowling, J.J. (1985) 'A modelling strategy for the smoothing of biomechanical data', in B. Jonsson (ed.), *Biomechanics X-B*, , Champaign, IL: Human Kinetics.

Fuller, J., Liu, L.J., Murphy, M.C. and Mann, R.W. (1997) 'A comparison of lower-extremity skeletal kinematics measured using skin- and pin-mounted markers', *Human Movement Science*, 16: 219–242.

Grabiner, M.D., Feuerbach, J.W., Lundin, T.M. and Davis, B.L. (1995) 'Visual guidance to force plates does not influence ground reaction force variability', *Journal of Biomechanics*, 28: 1115–1117.

Hall, M.G., Fleming, H.E., Dolan, M.J., Millbank, S.F.D. and Paul, J.P. (1996) 'Static in situ calibration of force plates', *Journal of Biomechanics*, 29: 659–665.

Hatze, H. (1980) 'A mathematical model for the computational determination of parameter values of anthropomorphic segments', *Journal of Biomechanics*, 13: 833–843.

Hatze, H. (1981) 'The use of optimally regularized Fourier series for estimating higher-order derivatives of noisy biomechanical data', *Journal of Biomechanics* 14: 13–18.

Kerwin, D.G. and Chapman, A.E. (1988) 'The frequency content of hurdling and running', in *Biomechanics in Sport*, London: The Institution of Mechanical Engineers.

Lanshammar, H. (1982) 'On precision limits for derivatives numerically calculated from noisy data', *Journal of Biomechanics*, 15: 459–470.

McCaw, S.T. and Devita, P. (1995) 'Errors in alignment of center of pressure and foot coordinates affect predicted lower extremity torques', *Journal of Biomechanics*, 28: 985–988.

Mungiole, M. and Martin, P.E. (1990) 'Estimating segment inertial properties: Comparison of magnetic resonance imaging with existing techniques', *Journal of Biomechanics*, 23: 1039–1046.

Rabuffetti, M., Ferrarin, M., Mazzoleni, P., Benvenuti, F. and Pedotti, A. (2003) 'Optimised procedure for the calibration of the force platform location', *Gait and Posture*, 17: 75–80.

Shannon, C.E. (1948) 'A mathematical theory of communication', *Bell Systems Technical Journal*, 27: 379–423.

Slepian, D. (1976) 'On bandwidth', *Proceedings of the IEEE*, 64: 292–300.

Veldpaus, F.E., Woltring, H.J. and Dortmans, L.J.M.G. (1988) 'A least-squares algorithm for the equiform transformation from spatial marker co-ordinates', *Journal of Biomechanics*, 21: 45–54.

Winter, D.A., Sidwall, H.G. and Hobson, D.A. (1974) 'Measurement and reduction of noise in kinematics of locomotion', *Journal of Biomechanics*, 7: 157–159.

Woltring, H.J. (1980) 'Planar control in multi-camera calibration for three-dimensional gait studies', *Journal of Biomechanics*, 13: 39–48.

Woltring, H.J. (1985) 'On optimal smoothing and derivative estimation from noisy displacement data in biomechanics', *Human Movement Science*, 4: 229–245.

Woltring, H.J. (1986) 'A Fortran package for generalized, cross-validatory spline smoothing and differentiation', *Advances in Engineering Software*, 8: 104–113.

Woltring, H.J. (1994) '3-D attitude representation of human joints: a standardization proposal', *Journal of Biomechanics*, 27: 1399–1414.

Woltring, H.J., Huiskes, R., de Lange, A. and Veldpaus, F.E. (1985) 'Finite centroid and helical axis estimation from noisy landmark measurements in the study of human joint kinematics', *Journal of Biomechanics*, 18: 379–389.

Wood, G.A. and Marshall, R.N. (1986) 'The accuracy of DLT extrapolation in three-dimensional film analysis', *Journal of Biomechanics*, 19: 781–785.

Yeadon, M.R. and Morlock, M. (1989) 'The appropriate use of regression equations for the estimation of segmental inertia parameters', *Journal of Biomechanics*, 27: 683–689.

CHAPTER 8

RESEARCH METHODS: SAMPLE SIZE AND VARIABILITY EFFECTS ON STATISTICAL POWER

David R. Mullineaux

INTRODUCTION

Most research in biomechanics involves the analysis of time-series data. In performing this analysis, several sequential and linked stages of proposing, conducting, analysing and reporting of research need to be performed (Mullineaux *et al.*, 2001). A key issue within each of these stages can be proposed. Firstly, the research question must be worthy, ethical and realistic. The research question should be used to try to outline how to propose, support or improve a theory. Secondly, the research design must be valid and use the best available methods. Thirdly, the data analysis must be accurate and meaningful. Lastly, the research must be interpreted and reported effectively. In planning a study, attention is often devoted to assessing statistical power. Power is affected by the research design, which in turn influences the accuracy of the statistical data produced. The aim of this chapter is to highlight factors affecting power, both through the research design and implementation of data transformations, while focusing on methods to explore and analyse time-series data.

STATISTICAL POWER

One of the main uses of statistics evident in the literature is 'statistical significance testing' of the null hypothesis. Essentially this application only provides the probability of the results when chance is assumed to have caused them, i.e. the null hypothesis is assumed to be true. Carver (1978, p. 383) refers to this as 'statistical rareness' where, for example, if $P < 0.05$ then obtaining a difference this large would be 'rare' and expected to occur less than 5% of the time as the null hypothesis is true. This single bit of information is used to identify whether the null hypothesis supports the data or not.

Statistical significance testing does not provide any other information, such as a description, reliability, validity, generalisability, effect authenticity or importance of the data. Despite this limited information, an over-reliance on statistical significance testing in research has prompted concern since early on in their use; Tyler, 1931 (p. 116) stated, '… differences which are statistically significant are not always socially important. The corollary is also true: differences which are not shown to be statistically significant may nevertheless be socially significant'. More recently, Lenth, 2001 (p. 1) stated, '… sample size may not be the main issue, that the real goal is to design a high-quality study'.

This recognised problem may suggest that statistical significance testing should not be used. However, this is unwise as scientific research is entrenched with the need for these statistics, and 'for scientists to abandon the textbook significance tests would be professional suicide' (Matthews, 1998, p. 24). Consequently, to reduce the impact of an over-reliance on statistical significance testing, the skill of the researcher is vital, requiring that he or she considers statistical power through, for example, carefully planning and implementing a research design; using various additional statistics to explore and describe data, such as descriptive statistics, effect size, confidence intervals, standard errors and reliability; and applying data transformations.

Statistical significance testing is encapsulated by the concept of 'statistical power', often simply referred to as 'power'. In essence, the research design and methods affect power, and power affects the outcome of the analysis – i.e. the statistical significance value. Power, 'the ability of a test to correctly reject a false null hypothesis' (Vincent, 1999, p. 138) is affected by factors in the research design, statistics and data, some of which have been summarised in Table 8.1.

In addition to setting the factors in Table 8.1 before the study, the researcher is also able to apply various solutions to the data obtained to help meet any assumptions. For instance, analytical solutions to replacing missing data, identifying and correcting for univariate and multivariate outliers, and correcting for violations of assumptions of linearity, normality and homoscedasticity can all be applied and would generally be expected to improve statistical power. Many of these solutions are described in textbooks; for example, common transformations to improve the normality of different data distributions have been described by Tabachnick and Fidell, 2001 (p. 82).

In addition to corrections for assumptions, decreasing the variability in the data can increase statistical power. Although increasing sample size is cited the most for increasing statistical power, reducing variability in the data has been considered more cost-effective (Shultz and Sands, 1995). Estimating the sample size is simple, and it is often used to meet many ethics committees' requirement that power is appropriately set *a-priori* so that estimates of the Type I and Type II error rates are acceptable for the planned study (the Type I error rate is the probability of incorrectly rejecting a null hypothesis as it is true; the Type II error rate is the probability of incorrectly accepting a null hypothesis as it is false). Decreasing variability has both simple solutions, such as using a more reliable measurement device or dependent variable, and complex ones,

Table 8.1   Research design, statistics and data factors affecting statistical power

Factor	Statistical power	
	Lower	Higher
Research design		
Type I error rate, alpha (α)	Small (e.g. 0.05)	Large (e.g. 0.10)
Type II error rate, beta (β)[a]	Large (e.g. 0.40)	Small (e.g. 0.20)
Sample size, *n*	Small	Large
Reliability of measurement	Poor	Good
Statistic		
Design	Between	Within
Tailed	Two	One (but power zero if incorrect)
Distribution assumed test	Non-normal	Normal
Distribution free test	Normal	Non-normal
Data[b]		
Effect size, ES	Small	Large
Mean difference	Small	Large
Variability	Large	Small

Notes:
[a]Typically set at 4 times α (Cohen, 1988) and used to calculate power $= (1 - \beta)^* 100$.
[b]Before the study estimates of ES determined from previous literature. In a simple form, ES is the ratio of the mean difference to variability.

such as applying a multiplicative scatter correction. An overview of methods to estimate sample size and decrease variability is provided below.

ESTIMATING SAMPLE SIZE

In recruiting participants for a study, the goal is to select a sample that is representative of the population. The sample statistics should therefore provide a reliable and unbiased predictor of the population parameter. In general, the probability of a biased sample increases as the sample size decreases; this increases the sampling error – the error in the estimate of a population parameter from a sample statistic. On this basis, tables have been developed to indicate the sample size (*n*) required for a given population size (*N*) which provide the variation, with known confidence, of the sample statistics from the population parameters (see Krejcie and Margan, 1970). Assuming that the results are to be based on a randomly selected sample and generalised to the population from which the sample was drawn, such tables are easy to use. On the basis of the three stages in sampling – define a population; identify a sampling frame; use a sampling technique – identifying the sampling frame that provides a list of all members of the population and subsequently indicates the population size is sometimes straightforward, as in listing the population of the top 100 middle distance runners, but more often difficult, such as identifying the population size of runners experiencing lower back pain. In this former example, based on a table in Krejcie and Margan, 1970, a sample of 80 of the top 100 middle distance runners would be required to identify the population parameters to within 5% with 90% confidence. Consequently, the relatively small sample sizes used in biomechanics presumably have a much smaller confidence in their representation of the population parameters, which may offer a partial explanation of any variation in sample statistics found between what appear to be similar studies. Nevertheless, often in a study the researcher is interested in assessing statistical significance, for example, whether differences between treatments can be attributable to chance at a specified statistical significance level. Consequently, alternative techniques are required to provide an estimate of the sample size when statistical significance is being used.

Selecting an appropriate sample size is principally related to achieving a desired statistical power. Methods of determining sample size with respect to statistical power are primarily based upon the interaction between four factors: sample size (n), effect size (ES), and the Type I (α) and II (β) error rates (see Table 8.1). These methods include using statistical formulas, tables, prediction equations and power software. Overall, the uses of these methods, examples of which are described in Box 8.1, are straightforward.

There are, however, issues that can limit the usefulness of the methods for performing a power analysis. Firstly, once a required sample size has been estimated, the practicality of implementing a study with a moderate or large sample size is difficult. In biomechanics research, sample sizes are often small owing to the complexity of biomechanical testing and its time-consuming, and thus expensive, methods. In the 1998 *Journal of Applied Biomechanics*, the sample size was reported to range from 3 to 67 (mean = 14.5; Mullineaux *et al.*, 2001). The ability to test greater numbers more efficiently is improving with technological advances, but large sample sizes will still be a rare phenomenon. This potentially introduces a bias of the sample not representing the population, such that statistical significance testing may have insufficient power, increasing the Type II error rate. Nevertheless, often in sport and exercise biomechanics, as the research question applies to smaller populations, for example the technique of elite performers, this may introduce a smaller bias than in research applicable to larger populations, such as ergonomics of industrial workers, and the high reliability of many of the measurement techniques will increase statistical power.

Secondly, these methods generally rely on the effect size being determined from previous literature, and using criterion values denoting what is a small, moderate or large effect. For example, effect sizes of 0.2, 0.5 and >0.8 represent small, moderate and large differences (Cohen, 1988), respectively, where a moderate difference is considered visible to an experienced researcher (Cohen, 1992, p. 156). Both determining the effect size from previous literature and using criterion values for effect size have been considered a major limitation of estimating power (Lenth, 2001). This was emphasised by Mullineaux *et al.*, 2001 (p. 749) in that effect size should consider 'what is an important difference theoretically, ethically, economically and practically, and considering whether the differences are bigger than limits identified for error, reliability and

Box 8.1   Examples of the use of four methods of power analysis for estimating sample size

Statistical formulae exist for some common tests, but not all. For the Independent *t*-test, $n = (2s^2(Z_\alpha + Z_\beta)^2)/\Delta^2$ (Eq. 1, Vincent, 1999, p. 142), where *s* is the estimated population standard deviation, Δ is the estimated difference between the two group means, and Z_α and Z_β are the *Z* scores on the normal curve for the desired Type I (α) and II (β) error rates, respectively. To determine Z_α and Z_β, tables of the area under the normal curve can be used, or more easily use the NORMSINV function in Excel (Microsoft Corporation, Redmond, WA). For example, the sample size for a two-tailed independent *t*-test, where $s = 8$, $\Delta = 7$, $\alpha = 0.05$ and $\beta = 0.20$, using $n = (2*s^2*(NORMSINV(\alpha/2) + NORMSINV(\beta))^2)/\Delta^2$ (Eq. 2) indicates 20 participants per group are required to achieve a power of 80% (i.e. $(1 - \beta)*100$; Eq. 3). Note, in equation 1, α is divided by 2 for the two-tailed test – if a one-tailed test is preferred then the required sample size would be 18 participants per group.

Tables, based on group size (*n*), effect size (ES), α, and β, have been developed for many tests. For example, based on effect sizes of small ($f = 0.10$), moderate ($f = 0.25$) and large ($f = 0.40$), and reading the table from Cohen (1998, pp. 315-316), to achieve an 80% power for a 1 way between ANOVA for 4 groups, $\alpha = 0.05$ and a moderate effect size (i.e. $f = 0.25$), the required sample size is 44 per group.

Prediction equations exist for several tests. These formulas are particularly helpful for repeated measures designs where formulas and tables are generally unavailable. For instance, Equation 4 can be used to determine the power (Ω) for the group main effect for a two group mixed ANOVA with α set to 0.05 (Park and Schutz, 1999, p. 259, where: *n* is sample size; *d* is effect size; *r* is mean correlation between the repeated measures; *q* is number of levels of the repeated measures factor). Setting up a spreadsheet to use these formulas is beneficial. Hence, to approximate the power to 0.80 (i.e. 80%) for $d = 0.6$, $r = 0.5$ and $q = 3$, the required sample size is 30. Note, the powers are different for the repeated measures factor (85%) and the interaction (50%), and these are determined using additional formulas.

$$\Omega = -0.00000442n^2 + 0.115/d^2 + 0.085\sqrt{n} - 0.785\sqrt{r} - 0.917/d - 2.066/\sqrt{n} - 0.329/q + 2.585 \text{ Eq. 4}$$

Power software is available, including some interactive web sites. For example, using the web page http://www.math.yorku.ca/SCS/Online/power/ (Friendly, 2003) and the example for the Table method above (i.e. where 44 participants were required per group for a one-way ANOVA, 4 groups, $\alpha = 0.05$ and moderate effect size), from this website an estimate of 40 participants per group is required. The website is set-up as follows:

- Number of levels of effect 'A' = 4 (i.e. the 4 factors of the one-way between ANOVA).
- Total number of levels of all other factors crossed with effect 'A' = 1 (i.e. 1 for a one-way ANOVA).
- Error level (alpha) for which you want power or sample size calculated = 0.05.
- Effect size(s) for which you want power or sample size calculated = 0.25 0.75 1.25 (note, in this web site these three values correspond to effect sizes of small, moderate and large).

variability analyses'. This is further supported by Hopkins *et al.*, 1999, who suggested that differences between elite performers are tiny and, as such, much smaller effect sizes might be meaningful in such circumstances. Alternatively, the researcher might decide on a particular effect size for the study being undertaken. For example, if the findings are to have real practical implications, then a large effect size of 0.8 might be chosen. But if the research is new, and the researcher feels it is important to detect any difference, even if small, then an effect size of 0.2 could be chosen (cited effect size values based on the definitions of Cohen, 1988).

Thirdly, the effect size is affected by many factors, some general ones of which are described in Table 8.1. For example, on-line motion capture systems are more reliable, although not necessarily more valid, than manual digitising. Greater reliability reduces variability, which in turn will increase the effect size. Consequently, estimates of the effect size from previous literature should factor in differences in methods, or acknowledge or recognise limitations in the work. Furthermore, it could simply be a problem that the information to estimate the effect size does not exist, as either no similar variables have previously been used or reported. Reporting means and standard deviations in abstracts for key variables is thus important as these provide the reader with data for a simple estimate of the effect size.

Although power is considered important by many authors (e.g. Howell, 1997), setting the sample size based on other issues both increases power and meets other statistical assumptions. For example, using a sample size of no less than 30 per group has been recommended when testing for differences between groups (Baumgartner and Strong, 1998) to increase the probability of a normal sampling distribution on the dependent variable, an assumption on which statistical tables, such as those of the t- and F-statistics, are based. In addition, specific statistical tests benefit from minimum sample sizes to improve the validity of the analysis. For example, a small ratio of the sample size (n) to the number of predictor variables (p) in regression analysis can cause problems. A small ratio can result in high correlations occurring by chance and the generality of the regression equation will be limited. The recommended $n{:}p$ ratio varies between authors, hence Mullineaux and Bartlett, 1997, proposed, as a rule of thumb, use at least 10:1 and, ideally, have between 20:1 and 40:1, where the largest ratio would be required for a stepwise multiple regression.

In addition to determining the sample size required on the basis of statistical grounds, consideration of other factors is important. For instance, estimating and minimising the attrition rate of participants from, for example, injury, absence or drop-out should be made. As well as losing participants during the study being time-consuming, it is also problematic as these participants may possess the principal characteristics that you may be most interested in studying. For example, in analysing the propensity of the elderly to hip fractures, the increased risks observed in some testing procedures may lead to hip fractures and, subsequently, the loss of the participant. Consequently, it is important to implement a design with some compromise over the 'desired' protocol to minimise attrition. For example, reducing the intensity of the protocol, the number of testing sessions or the duration of the experiment may be suitable. Also, it is important to provide an adequate extrinsic motivation – to explain 'what is in it' for them – and to interact with the participants. Possible methods to reduce attrition include sampling participants carefully, keeping participants informed, collecting data efficiently, acting courteously and professionally at all times, talking to your participants, making the testing interesting, explaining the results, minimising potentially embarrassing environments – such as not testing in a publicly visible laboratory, and keeping a clean and tidy laboratory. However, some participant attrition, missing data or removing outlier scores should be expected. The resulting missing data should be evaluated, first for patterns – for example outlier scores may be associated with a particular trait and, therefore, may be important – and then to ascertain whether the data should be replaced. Replacing these values is advantageous as it retains participants in the dataset and, consequently, the degrees of freedom remains larger thus increasing statistical power. In contrast, there are always limitations in replacing missing values. These will not be covered here, although using prior knowledge, mean scores, regression analysis, expectation maximisation and multiple imputation are explained as methods of replacing missing data (see Tabachnick and Fidell, 2001, p. 60). Another simple method is that the missing value should equal the row mean plus the column mean minus the grand mean (Winer *et al.*, 1991).

In summary, if sample sizes are small then generalising the results to a larger population should be viewed with caution. When statistical significance testing is being used to determine whether chance can account for the difference, then power analyses are beneficial in choosing an appropriate sample size, but power analyses must not be used *post hoc* to help explain results (Lenth, 2001). Power analyses can be problematic, however, in that they require data from previous literature that may not necessarily be of adequate quality or even address the variables of interest. In addition, these analyses principally require sample size to be altered, whereas other factors influencing statistical power can be used, some of which are described in Table 8.1. These may provide the means to implement more efficient experimental designs, for example, powerful yet without large sample sizes. Such additional factors to increase statistical power are considered in the next section.

REDUCING VARIABILITY

In biomechanics, large variability often exists between individuals, which can arise through the methods and the population being investigated. Reducing this variability provides a key method for increasing statistical power. Variability can be reduced through the research design and methods by, for example, using a more reliable measure, averaging several trials, removing noise through filtering, or correcting for the violation of statistical assumptions. In addition, reducing variability by catering for the individuality in the data is also effective; this may be particularly important in 'elite' and 'injured' populations owing to their uniqueness and small sample size that make generalisations difficult. The main method of removing systematic differences between individuals is by normalising the data, either as a ratio or through an offset. Alternatively, if inferential statistics are not required then simply providing descriptive statistics is an effective way of reporting the results, as has been provided in the past (e.g. Burden *et al.*, 1998). Several of these approaches will be expanded upon.

Ratio normalisation

Ratio normalisation is underpinned by the assumption that a theoretical and statistical relationship exists between the dependent variable and a covariate.

When this relates to an energetic variable as the dependent variable and a body dimensions as the covariate then normalisation is a form of scaling known as allometry (Schmidt-Nielsen, 1984). Applying allometry is generally beneficial as it is able to cater for non-linear relationships, although the result may be linear. There has been a renewed interest in this topic applied to humans, but scientific literature on allometry dating back to 1838 has been cited (see Winter and Nevill, 2001). Generally, allometry is appropriate for identifying the extent to which performance differences are attributable to differences in size or to differences in qualitative characteristics of the body's tissues and structures (Winter and Nevill, 2001, p. 275). In addition, as allometry can cater for non-linear relationships, it is suitable for addressing the non-isometric and isometric changes in dimensions with growth (Tanner, 1989). It is important that such analyses are underpinned by theory. Dimensionality theory offers one possible theoretical basis for an allometric scaling analysis.

Dimensionality theory is underpinned by the Système International d'Unités that comprises seven base units (mass, length, time, electric current, temperature, amount of substance and luminous intensity). From these seven units all other units, such as area, volume, density, force, pressure, energy, power and frequency, can be derived. Often for convenience, these units are renamed; for example, the units of force – $kg\,m\,s^{-2}$ – are denoted as newtons (N). Dimensionality theory can be used for two main purposes (Duncan, 1987): dimensional homogeneity and dimensional analysis. Dimensional homogeneity can be used to check that an equation is correct by partitioning both sides of an equation into their base units. If the units on both sides are partitioned into the same base units then the equation is correct. Dimensional analysis can be used to predict the relationship between different dimensions as a means to provide a theoretical foundation for a research study, such as between several continuous variables.

When there are two continuous variables (y and x), they can be scaled with each other in many forms, three of which are common: ratio standard ($y = bx$), linear regression ($y = a + bx$) and non-linear ($y = ax^b$), where a and b are constants. The use of each of these scaling techniques should be dictated by theory, although the theory is not always obvious. In addition, the mathematics of, and the assumptions for, a scaling technique delimit their use theoretically and statistically. For example, non-linear scaling may be appropriate for data that are not necessarily linear and, theoretically, requires a zero intercept and contains multiplicative error about the regression. The opposite assumptions are made in ratio standard or linear regression scaling analyses in that the data are linear, the intercept is not fixed at zero and the error is additive. Many of these assumptions are explained in textbooks (e.g. Tabachnick and Fidell, 2001) and are illustrated in a paper in which these assumptions also underpin some repeated-measures reliability statistics (Mullineaux et al., 1999).

Another benefit of scaling is that it provides the data normalisation that removes the effects of a covariate. An additional benefit is that more than one independent variable, including one dummy variable as a dichotomous independent variable coded as 0 and 1 can be included in a multiple scaling analysis. This will increase the explained variance and reduce the effect of extraneous variables, but more statistical assumptions, such as multicollinearity, need to be checked to validate the analysis. This has been applied in an allometric scaling analysis to determine a difference between the sexes in left ventricular heart mass (Batterham *et al.*, 1997). Simple scaling (e.g. $y = ax^b$) is easy to perform, but when there is more than one independent variable in non-linear scaling, for example, $y = ax_1^b + cx_2^d$, where x_1 and x_2 are independent variables, and c and d are constants, it is easier to use a log-log transformation in combination with multiple linear regression analyses. As the data are non-linear, where the error is often multiplicative, then the first log transformation generally linearises the relationship, alters the error to being additive and improves the normality distribution of the data. These are all necessary assumptions underpinning a linear regression scaling analysis.

In scaling analyses, providing a theory that supports the relationship identified can be difficult. In particular, this is difficult in data analyses that routinely use ratio standard or linear regression scaling; yet their use is still common. For example, normalisation to lean body mass for ground reaction forces (Raftopoulos *et al.*, 2000), limb length for stride length (Cham and Redfern, 2002), and maximal isometric contractions for electromyographic data (Pullinen *et al.*, 2002) have been used. A further limitation of ratio standard and linear regression scaling has been proposed in that extrapolation beyond the data range should be avoided as this would not generally meet the zero intercept assumption (Batterham *et al.*, 1997). However, this caution may also need to be applied to allometrically scaled relationships, as the assumption of a zero intercept is often beyond the data range that could be tested empirically. A further consideration is that although scaling is often used to remove the effect of a covariate (x) on the dependent variable (y), alternative methods are available. Nevertheless, non-linear and, specifically, allometric scaling has been demonstrated as superior to both ratio-normalisation and analysis of covariance (ANCOVA) in removing the effects of a covariate on the dependent variable (Winter and Neville, 2001). To confirm that the effects of a covariate have been removed through normalisation, a correlation between the dependent variable and the newly normalised data should be close to zero (Batterham *et al.*, 1997). If this correlation is not near zero, or at least is not smaller than the correlation between the dependent variable and the covariate, then the normalisation has been inappropriate and may have introduced more variability into the data that will decrease statistical power.

One method of providing theoretical support for a suitable scaling factor is to use dimensionality analysis. For instance, force is proportional to mass; mass is proportional to volume; volume to the power of 0.67 equals cross-sectional area (CSA). Consequently, CSA and force are proportional to mass to the power of 0.67. Empirically, using dynamometry, it has been recommended that muscle force be normalised to body mass to the power of 0.67 (Jaric, 2002). In another example, to cater for participants of different sizes, ground reaction forces are often normalised to body mass (Duffey *et al.*, 2000), although it has been suggested that normalising ground reaction forces to lean body mass is more appropriate (Raftopoulos *et al.*, 2000). A comparison of normalising ground reaction force and loading rates to body mass to different power exponents has been performed (Mullineaux *et al.*, 2006). Ground reaction forces were appropriately normalised using body mass to the power of 1, linearly; but for loading rates a power exponent of 0.67 was generally better. Consequently linear normalisation of loading rates may inappropriately favour heavier participants because the proposed 0.67 power exponent would result in a greater relative reduction in loading rates for heavier than for lighter participants. However, the correct allometrically scaled relationships between energetic variables, such as ground reaction and muscle forces, with body dimensions, such as body mass and CSA, requires further investigation.

The ratio normalisation methods mentioned above can be classified as a 'simple ratio' type. More complex methods also exist which include standard normal variate transformation – normalise to the standard deviation of the data – and derivative normalising – normalise to the magnitude of the first derivative of the data. The 'simple ratio' methods change the magnitude of the data, but complex methods may also change the shape of the time-series data. Further details on these complex methods will not be covered. In the next subsection, an alternative form of normalisation using offsets is covered. Some of the benefits and limitations that are further expanded upon with regard to offset-normalisation below may well be appropriate to consider with the ratio-normalisation techniques covered here.

Offset normalisation

Normalising data using offsets can also be classified as simple and complex. Simple offsets commonly include subtracting the difference between the individual and the group mean for a defined measure. The measure may include a value within the data – such as the initial value, value at a key instant, the minimum, or the mean – or external to the data, such as a morphological value or criterion value. More complex methods include detrending, Fourier transform and multiplicative scatter correction. Detrending involves fitting a polynomial regression to the data, which is then used as the defined measure. The Fourier transform, that is using the waveform of sum of weighted sines and cosines as the defined measure, has been used to correct skin marker movement in kinematic analyses of horses (van Weeren et al., 1992). The use of multiplicative scatter correction, using the linear regression coefficients of the mean data as the defined measure, has been demonstrated for reducing variability in kinematic data (Mullineaux et al., 2004).

As with all techniques, offset normalisations can be used in various ways. Multiplicative scatter correction contains additive (intercept of the regression) and multiplicative (slope of the regression) elements that can individually or, as recommended, both be removed (Næs et al., 2002). Generally offset-normalising reduces the variability in the data, and the shape of the data is retained with the simple offsets, but the shape is often altered with more complex methods.

In biomechanics, the use of offset normalising may be beneficial, particularly for kinematic data, owing to variations in morphology that produce differences in limb lengths and standing angles. Correcting for some of these variations in morphology and kinematics may be important not only to improve statistical power but also to assist in a valid interpretation of the data. In equine biomechanics, some simple offset normalisation techniques have been applied to cater for variations in morphology, including using a joint's standing angle (Back *et al.*, 1994), angle at hoof impact (Holmström *et al.*, 1994; although this was incorrectly referred to as a multiplicative scatter correction) and mean trace (Degueurce *et al.*, 1997).

Assuming the data have been normalised to the same time of 101 points, the simple offset formulae is $New_{ki} = Original_{ki} + (D_{MEAN} - D_k)$. Hence, to obtain the simple offset normalised data (New_{ki}), the non-normalised data ($Original_{ki}$) for each individual (k) at each per cent of time (i) needs to be summed with the difference between the defined measures of the group mean (D_{MEAN}) and each individual's mean (D_k). As an example of a complex offset normalisation, the formula for a multiplicative scatter correction (MSC) is $MSC = Original_{ki} - a_k/b_k$, where the linear regression for the entire stride ($y_k = a_k x + b_k$) between the mean group (x) and each individual (y_k) provides the constants a_k and b_k (Næs *et al.*, 2002).

Comparison of three simple offset normalisations – mean, initial and standing angles, and one complex normalisation – multiplicative scatter correction, has been provided by Mullineaux *et al.*, 2004. Several key features emerged from these normalisations.

- Choosing a defined measure external to the data was recommended. Although this does not reduce the variability the most, defined measures within the data result in 'local' variability reductions. For instance, using the initial value resulted in the variability reducing to zero at the beginning of the data, which was the instant the foot made ground contact.
- The complex offset of a multiplicative scatter correction reduced the variability the most. However, it was not recommended as the shape of each participant's trace was altered which distorted within-individual data comparisons.
- Offset normalisation reduced the variability sufficiently to increase power and result in more variables becoming significant. Care was recommended in the interpretation of the results as mean angle changes pre- and post-intervention of only $1°$ were found to be statistically significantly different, which was considered lower than the error limit of the data collection.
- Normalisation improved the normality distribution assumption of the data in their study, although it was recommended that following any data transformation the normality distribution should be checked.
- Reporting variability for both sets of data, pre- and post-normalisation, was recommended so as to enable comparisons between studies.

Analysing multiple trials

Two main methods of reducing variability using ratio and offset normalisations have been covered above. An additional method of reducing variability that is becoming more common in biomechanics is to collect multiple trials and to use the average score. Issues on this have been covered in detail elsewhere, which include a statistical rationale for using the 'average' instead of the 'best' trial (e.g. Kroll, 1957) and, as a simple recommendation, that at least three trials should be used as a compromise between statistical issues and practicality (see Mullineaux *et al.*, 2001). This overcomes the limitation that one trial may not be representative of the performer's 'normal' technique (Bates *et al.*, 1992).

As averaging trials is arguably problematic, as it essentially creates a mythical trial, it is possible to analyse these multiple trials in a nested analysis of variance (ANOVA). In many software packages these analyses are not straightforward to perform or analyse and, more importantly, it is unclear how many trials should be used. This affects the statistical power; hence recommendations on using nested analyses still needs investigating. However, another approach is to use single-individual analyses in which the multiple trials by a single participant provide the individual measures in statistical analyses. Generally, between-group statistics are used (Bates, 1996) as, otherwise, trial order influences the statistical significance obtained. Nevertheless, if trial order is relevant or justified, as when matching by trial order or ranking trials from worst to best, statistical power can be increased by using a within-group statistic. Single-individual analyses overcome another potential limitation of group analyses: if similarities in performers' techniques do not exist then the data may represent a mythical 'average' performer (Dufek *et al.*, 1995). Where similarities do not exist, then this decreases statistical power. Examples of the application of single-individual analyses include Hreljac, 1998, and Wheat *et al.*, 2003. These analyses can also provide 'baseline' variability for a participant that can be analysed in longitudinal studies. The use of multiple trials also paves the way for analysing variability itself, which is covered in the next section.

ANALYSING VARIABILITY IN TIMES-SERIES DATA

Rather than reducing variability for statistical purposes, it can be meaningful to analyse and discuss variability in light of its importance in the successful control and outcomes of movement. In analysing variability – the departure from the central score – greater measures have been viewed as indicative of poor technique (Davids *et al.*, 1997), functional in producing the desired outcome (Arutyunyan *et al.*, 1968) and reducing injury risk (Hamill *et al.*, 1999; Heiderscheit *et al.*, 1999; 2000). Conversely, for example, less variability has been viewed as an indication of injury (Peham *et al.*, 2001). In particular, variability can provide a measure of coordination – the functional link between the muscles and joints used to produce the desired performance or outcome. Various methods exist to quantify variability.

With respect to kinematic data, which provide the researcher with a simplified representation of human movement, often discrete values are reported for single variables or combinations of several variables, such as the ratio of hip to knee angles. These discrete values may be for key instants, such as the start of a movement, a descriptive statistic such as the minimum or maximum, or representative of the entire movement such as the mean. Several methods are available for quantifying variability within these discrete values. Five methods, namely standard deviation (SD), root mean square difference (RMSD), 95% confidence intervals (95% CI), per cent coefficient of variation (%CV) and per cent RMSD (%RMSD), have been considered previously (Mullineaux *et al.*, 2001). Assuming that RMSD is calculated based on the mean score providing the criterion value (although independent criterion scores can be used, for example, in an error analysis) then, if the mean, standard deviation and sample size are provided, all of these methods are determinable from each other, facilitating comparisons between different measures used in the literature. In general, if $n > 3$, then 95% CI provide the smallest measure, followed by the RMSD and then the SD.

The analysis of discrete values provides an easily obtainable measure of a performance. However, the reporting of discrete values alone has been criticised as these fail to capture the dynamics of movement (e.g. Baumann, 1992). The dynamics of movement can qualitatively be assessed from graphical plots of single or multiple variables. Three main graphical representations exist: variable-time graphs (time series), variable-variable or angle-angle plots and phase-planes. If multiple trials are plotted, then, in addition to qualitatively assessing the patterns of movement, variability can be assessed. As human movement is complex, analysing variability using multiple variables may provide the most comprehensive information (Mullineaux and Wheat, 2002). Multiple variables are, or can be, presented in all three of these graphical plots and used to assess variability over the entire kinematic trace provided two or more trials are plotted. Each of these plots is used differently. To illustrate these plots, the knee and hip angles for three trials of a non-injured, male participant running at 3 m s^{-1} are used in Figures 8.1 to 8.8. With many of these techniques, it is necessary that the trials are of the same length. Consequently, these trials were normalised to 101 data points, which is also beneficial as it facilitates discussing per cent of time throughout the movement and it is easy to scale the time axis, i.e. to scale time from 0 to 100% of the overall movement.

Firstly, the variable-time graph of the knee and hip angles for three trials is presented in Figure 8.1. In the anatomical standing position, the knee is at 180° (flexion is positive) and the hip is at 0° (thigh segment to the vertical; flexion is positive; hyper-extension is negative). These two variables have been combined as a ratio of the hip to the knee angles (see Figure 8.2; left axis). The ratio of the two variables at each instant over the trials can be used to calculate the variability in the data. For instance, using the RMSD, with the mean as the criterion value, variability at each instance in the running cycle is presented in Figure 8.2 (right axis).

Secondly, the angle-angle plot of the knee and hip are presented in Figure 8.3. To quantify the variability in these data, vector coding can be applied (Tepavac and Field-Fote, 2001). Vector coding may be applicable to data that are not necessarily linearly related, as is assumed in cross-correlations – see later. To vector code from the angle-angle plot, determine the vector between each consecutive data point to obtain an angle and magnitude, and repeat this for each trial. At each time, determine the mean angle and mean magnitude across the trials. The product of the means of the angles

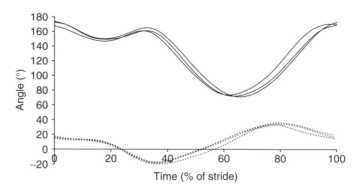

Figure 8.1 Angles for knee (solid lines) and hip (dashed lines) for three trials of a healthy, male participant running at 3 m s^{-1}. In the anatomical standing position, the knee is at 180° (flexion positive) and the hip is at 0° (thigh segment to the vertical; flexion positive; hyper-extension negative). Key events are right foot contact at 0% and 100%, and right foot off at 40%

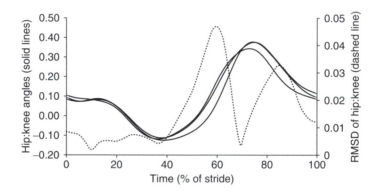

Figure 8.2 Ratio of the hip to the knee angles for three trials of a healthy, male participant running at 3 m s^{-1} (left axis), and using the mean score as the criterion the RMSD of these three trials (right axis). First 40% is right foot stance phase

and magnitudes provides the coefficient of correspondence (r). Together, this coefficient represents a summary of the angle (shape) and magnitude (size) of the trials, the plot of which indicates the variability throughout the movement (see Figure 8.4). The coefficient of correspondence varies from 0 (maximum variability) to 1 (no variability).

Thirdly, a phase-plane can be used to calculate variability using the continuous relative phase standard deviation (CRPsd; Hamill *et al.*, 1999; 2000; Kurz and Stergiou, 2002). A phase-plane represents the angular velocity of a variable plotted against its angle (see Figure 8.5). From this plot, the phase angle is calculated as the angle between the horizontal axis and the line from the origin to a data point. The difference between the phase angles between the two joints at corresponding time intervals throughout the entire cycle provides the relative phase angle or continuous relative phase (CRP; see Figure 8.6).

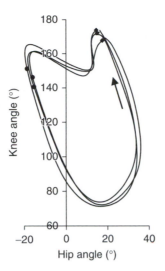

Figure 8.3 Knee–hip angle-angle diagram for three trials of a healthy, male participant running at 3 m s^{-1}. Heel strike (♦), toe off (•) and direction (arrow) indicated

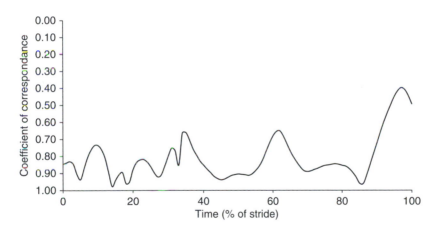

Figure 8.4 Coefficient of correspondence (*r*) determined using vector coding (Tepavac and Field-Fote, 2001) of three trials of the knee–hip angle-angle data for a healthy, male participant running at 3 m s^{-1}. The coefficient ranges from maximal variability (*r* = 0) to no variability (*r* = 1). First 40% is right foot stance phase

The standard deviation in the CRP provides the CRPsd (Figure 8.7), which illustrates the variability throughout the movement. The CRPsd, derived from the CRP that has principally been used as a direct measure of coordination, indirectly measures coordination through variability.

It is more complicated to calculate CRP than either the RMSD or vector coding, which has resulted in more papers addressing assumptions, methods and interpretation of CRP. In simple and sinusoidal movements CRP is considered

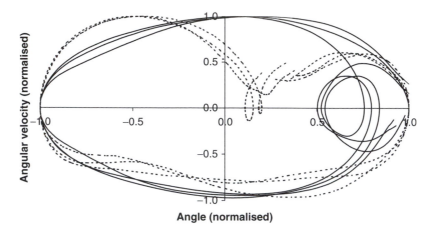

Figure 8.5 Phase-plane of the knee (solid lines) and hip (dashed lines) angles for three trials of a healthy, male participant running at 3 m s⁻¹. Angular velocity is normalised to the maximum value across trials (hence 0 represents zero angular velocity), and angle is normalised to the range within trials (i.e. −1 represents minimum, and +1 represents maximum value)

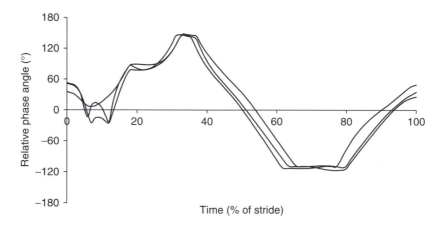

Figure 8.6 Continuous relative phase between the hip and knee angles of three trials of a healthy, male participant running at 3 m s⁻¹. Phase-plane angle (φ) used in the range of $0° \leq \varphi \leq 180°$. First 40% is right foot stance phase

to provide a good indication of two joints being in-phase (CRP = 0°) or anti-phase (out of phase; CRP = 180°; Hamill *et al.*, 2000). For more complex motions, such as in running, despite qualitatively similar phase-planes for the hip and knee, it has been concluded that CRP provided little information about the coordination between these two joints (Mullineaux and Wheat, 2002). This was principally attributable to the violation of the assumption of a sinusoidal distribution, requiring that a transformation be applied. To address this issue, normalising for the period of oscillation has been used (Peters *et al.*, 2003), and the authors also proposed sophisticated transforms such as

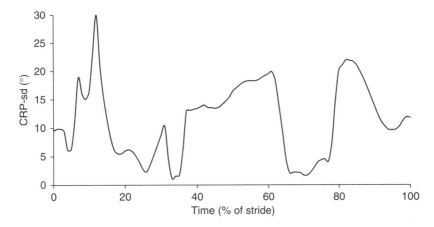

Figure 8.7 Continuous relative phase standard deviation (CRP-sd) in the three CRP angles between the hip and knee angles for three trials of a healthy, male participant running at 3 m s^{-1}. First 40% is right foot stance phase

the Hilbert Transform, non-linear methods, and interpolation of positional data as alternative methods to account for the violation of the sinusoidal distribution. Consequently, in calculating CRP various decisions need to be made, all of which will radically alter the results. These include which frequency transformation above to use, what component phase angle (φ) definition to use – often in the range $0° \leq \varphi \leq 180°$ – and how the data should be normalised. Various methods for normalising the data have been highlighted (see Hamill *et al.*, 2000; e.g. normalise angular velocity to 1 as the maximum of each trial, or to the maximum of all trials), which may improve the one-to-one ratio assumption. In contrast, as the arc tangent is used to calculate the component phase angle, it has been considered that this will account for differences in amplitudes between segments and, as such, no normalisation is required (Kurz and Stergiou, 2002).

In directly measuring coordination, it is possible to base this on only one trial, whereas measuring coordination indirectly through variability requires two or more trials. In addition to CRP as a direct measure of coordination, cross-correlation determined from angle-angle plots is also available. Cross-correlations provide a linear correlation coefficient between two sets of time-series data where one variable has a time lag introduced (Amblard *et al.*, 1994). A summary of recommendations for the use of cross-correlations have been made previously (Mullineaux *et al.*, 2001). These include that, as high correlation coefficients can occur for non-linear data, the linearity assumption across the entire data range should be checked visually by plotting one variable with no time lag against the other variable with its time lag introduced. Previously it has been demonstrated that the relationship between the hip and knee in running was linear at times but non-linear at other times (Mullineaux and Wheat, 2002). Potentially, analysing the data in phases, as has been performed previously (Hamill *et al.*, 1999), may be possible, and applying a linear transformation to the non-linear phase of the movement may improve the cross-correlational data analysis.

The techniques mentioned so far (listed in Table 8.2) have mainly been described for calculating a measure at each instant throughout the movement cycle. Many of these methods can also be used by taking an average of these measures across the entire cycle to provide an overall measure of the variability across the entire movement. In addition to these techniques, another measure provides this overall measure of variability simply; based on an angle-angle plot, the normalised root mean square difference (NoRMS) can be calculated, a technique which has been covered in depth elsewhere (see Sidaway et al., 1995; Mullineaux et al., 2001).

In summary, analysis of variability can be performed using various techniques. These tend to provide different 'qualitative' findings, as the periods of small and large variability may be used to infer any coordination strategies that vary between the techniques (see Figure 8.8; solid lines). In addition, the results are also difficult to compare quantitatively (see Table 8.2). The choice

Table 8.2 Statistical analyses available for quantifying variability and, consequently coordination, in two or more trials, across the entire cycle or as an overall measure for the entire cycle. The examples relate to three trials of a healthy, male participant running at 3 m s^{-1} (see Figures 8.1 to 8.7)

Basis	Technique (recommended reading)	Example Output[a]	
		Entire cycle	Overall
Variable-time graph (e.g. Figures 8.1, 8.2, left axis)	95%CI, SD, RMSD, %CV and %RMSD of a variable or ratio of variables (Mullineaux et al., 2001)	Figure 8.2 (right axis; RMSD of a ratio of 2 variables)	0.03
Angle-angle plot (e.g. Figure 8.3)	Vector coding (Tepavac and Field-Fote, 2001)	Figure 8.4	0.81[b]
	NoRMS (Sidaway et al., 1995; Mullineaux et al., 2001)	N/A	4.2%
	Cross-correlation, r (Amblard et al., 1994; Mullineaux et al., 2001)	N/A	0.83[c]
	Cross-correlation, time lag (Amblard et al., 1994; Mullineaux et al., 2001)*	N/A	−18%[c]
Phase plane (e.g. Figure 8.5)	Continuous Relative Phase, CRP (Hamill et al., 2000)[d]	Figure 8.6	N/A
	CRP standard deviation, CRPsd (Hamill et al., 2000)	Figure 8.7	7.6°

Notes:
[a]N/A indicates output not available from the technique.
[b]Data are a product of magnitude and angle components, both of which can be analysed independently.
[c]Average presented of the three trials for r (0.827; 0.830; 0.784) and the time lag (−17%; −18%; −17%; negative value indicates the hip moves before the knee). Calculated using SPSS 11.5.0 for Windows (SPSS, Chicago, IL).
[d]Provides a phase angle, which is a measure of coordination and not variability.

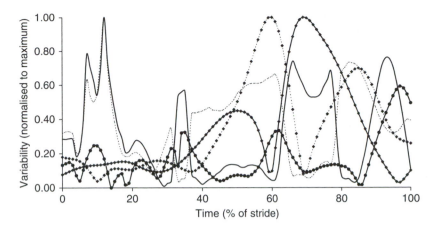

Figure 8.8 Quantification of variability in hip and knee angles for three trials of a healthy, male participant running at 3 m s^{-1} using vector coding (•), RMSD (♦) and continuous relative phase standard deviation (no symbol) for, when in the anatomical standing position, the hip is 0° (solid lines) and hip is 180° (dashed lines). Note, vector coding does not change with the hip angle definition. First 40% of time is the right foot stance phase

of which approach to use may depend on meeting underpinning assumptions, ease of use and interpretation, ability to compare to previous literature, and the preference of the researcher. Some comparisons in the literature include, for example, that cross-correlations were considered to provide a more meaningful measure of coordination than CRP (Mullineaux and Wheat, 2002). It was considered that a transformation technique might improve the assumptions for CRP, but that the greater data processing might not be warranted, as this could make the calculation and interpretation too complicated. A further consideration is that only vector coding, compared with RMSD and CRPsd, was found to provide the same results when the angle definition of the hip was altered. The definition of full extension was changed from 0° to 180°, as demonstrated in Figure 8.8 (compare solid with dashed lines). Consequently, as vector coding is the only reliable measure that is not dependent on the variable definition, and is simple to calculate, it may prove to be the most suitable measure for quantifying variability; however, other measures may become more viable through further development or standardisation.

REPORTING A STUDY

Reporting research effectively facilitates the dissemination of knowledge and subsequent advancement of science. A key feature in reporting research is to work within the pressure on space. In this chapter, which has focused on a small area of research methods, many factors have been highlighted that can affect results and consequently the meaning of data. For instance, angle definitions alter measures of variability and the method of treating trials affects statistical power. But, for example, in 20% of a selection of biomechanical papers the method of treating trials was unclear (Mullineaux *et al.*, 2001). Nevertheless, in combination with the other chapters of this book, it is suggested that you aim to:

- Report sufficient details to enable the reader to understand the theoretical underpinning of the research question, use the findings to support future research, replicate the study and interpret the findings.
- Cite references to standard procedures and statistical analyses, as throughout this chapter.
- Provide details on the defined population, sampling frame and sampling method, and report the sample characteristics.
- Outline the research design, including the timing, number and sequence of measurements, and provide details on trial sizes used and method of treating trials.
- Clarify methods, such as calibration procedures, to control for experimental errors.
- Address the reliability of the measurements.
- Provide informative results, particularly descriptive statistics as they provide simple data of practical value. Also reporting these in the abstract for key variables is beneficial as it allows the reader to perform a simple power analysis.
- Justify the level of inferential statistical significance (α) and probability values (P), and report an *a-priori* statistical power analysis and exact P values in the results.
- Justify the statistical analyses used.
- Report assessments and corrections applied to the assumptions of statistical tests.
- Use effect size statistics to supplement, or supplant, significance tests.
- Establish and quantify uncertainties in the data.
- Present information in the most appropriate format either in a chart, if a visual inspection is required, or a table, if exact values are important; duplication should be avoided.
- Focus the report on the research question that was addressed, the underlying theory, previous related research, the importance of the results of the study and how they contribute to existing knowledge, and assess the limitations of the study.
- List references accurately.

REFERENCES

Amblard, B., Assaiante, C., Lekhel, H. and Marchand, A.R. (1994) 'A statistical approach to sensorimotor strategies: conjugate cross-correlations', *Journal of Motor Behavior*, 26: 103–112.

Arutyunyan, G.H., Gurfinkel, V.S. and Mirskii, M.L. (1968) 'Investigation of aiming at a target', *Biophysics*, 13: 536–538.

Back, W., Barneveld, A., Bruin, G., Schamhardt, H.C. and Hartman, W. (1994) 'Kinematic detection of superior gait quality in young trotting Warmbloods', *The Veterinary Quarterly*, 16S2: 91–96.

Bates, B.T. (1996) 'Single subject methodology: an alternative approach', *Medicine and Science in Sports and Exercise*, 28: 631–638.

Bates, B.T., Dufek, J.S. and Davis, H.P. (1992) 'The effect of trial size on statistical power', *Medicine and Science in Sports and Exercise*, 24: 1059–1068.

Batterham, A.M., George, K.P. and Mullineaux, D.R. (1997) 'Allometric scaling of left ventricular mass and body dimensions in males and females', *Medicine and Science in Sports and Exercise*, 29: 181–186.

Baumann, W. (1992) Perspectives in methodology in biomechanics of sport, in R. Rodano, G. Ferrigno and G. Santambrogio (eds), *Proceedings of the Xth Symposium of the International Society of Biomechanics in Sports* (pp. 97–104), Milan, Italy: Edi Ermes.

Baumgartner, T.A. and Strong, C.H. (1998) *Conducting and Reading Research in Health and Human Performance*, Boston, MA: McGraw-Hill.

Burden, A.M., Grimshaw, P.N. and Wallace, E.S. (1998) 'Hip and shoulder rotations during the golf swing of sub-10 handicap players', *Journal of Sports Sciences*, 16: 165–176.

Carver, R.P. (1978) 'The case against statistical significance testing', *Harvard Educational Review*, 48: 378–399.

Cham, R. and Redfern, M.S. (2002) 'Changes in gait when anticipating slippery floors', *Gait and Posture*, 15: 159–171.

Cohen, J. (1988) *Statistical Power Analysis for the Behavioural Sciences*, Hillsdale, NJ: Lawrence Erlbaum.

Cohen, J. (1992) 'A power primer', *Psychological Bulletin*, 112: 155–159.

Davids, K., Bennett, S.J., Handford, C.H., Jolley, L. and Beak, S. (1997) Acquiring coordination in interceptive actions: an ecological approach, in R. Lidor and M. Bar-Eli (eds), *Innovations in Sport Psychology: Linking Theory and Practice* (pp. 227–229), Netanya, Israel: International Society of Sport Psychology.

Degueurce, C., Pourcelot, P., Audigié, F., Denoix, J.M. and Geiger, D. (1997) 'Variability of the limb joint patterns of sound horses at trot', *Equine Veterinary Journal*, 23S: 89–92.

Dufek, J.S., Bates, B.T., James, C.J. and Stergiou, N. (1995) 'Interactive effects between group and single-subject response patterns', *Human Movement Science*, 14: 301–323.

Duffey, M.J., Martin, D.F., Cannon, D.W., Craven, T. and Messier, S.P. (2000) 'Etiologic factors associated with anterior knee pain in distance runners', *Medicine and Science in Sports and Exercise*, 32: 1825–1832.

Duncan, T. (1987) *Physics: A Textbook for Advanced Level Students*, London: John Murray.

Friendly, M. (2003) 'Power analysis for ANOVA designs' *http://www.math.yorku.ca/SCS/Online/power/*, (accessed 16 October 2004).

Hamill, J., Haddad, M. and McDermott, W.J. (2000) 'Issues in quantifying variability from a dynamical systems perspective', *Journal of Applied Biomechanics*, 16: 407–418.

Hamill, J., van Emmerik, R.E.A., Heiderscheit, B.C. and Li, L. (1999) 'A dynamical systems approach to lower extremity running injuries', *Clinical Biomechanics*, 14: 297–308.

Heiderscheit, B.C. (2000) 'Movement variability as a clinical measure for locomotion', *Journal of Applied Biomechanics*, 16: 419–427.

Heiderscheit, B.C., Hamill, J. and van Emmerik, R.E.A. (1999) 'Q angle influences on the variability of lower extremity coordination', *Medicine and Science in Sports and Exercise*, 31: 1313–1319.

Holmström, M., Fredricson, I. and Drevemo, S. (1994) 'Biokinematic differences between riding horses judged as good and poor at the trot', *Equine Veterinary Journal*, 17S: 51–56.

Hopkins, W.G., Hawley, J.A. and Burke, L.M. (1999) 'Design and analysis of research on sport performance enhancement', *Medicine and Science in Sports and Exercise*, 31: 472–485.

Howell, D.C. (1997) *Statistical Methods for Psychology*, Belmont, CA: Duxbury Press.

Hreljac, A. (1998) 'Individual effects on biomechanical variables during landing in tennis shoes with varying midsole density', *Journal of Sports Sciences*, 16: 531–537.

Jaric, S. (2002) 'Muscle strength testing: use of normalisation for body size', *Sports Medicine*, 32: 615–631.

Krejcie, R.V. and Margan, D.W. (1970) 'Determining sample size for research activities', *Education and Psychological Measurement*, 30: 607–610.

Kroll, W. (1957) 'Reliability theory and research decision in selection of a criterion score', *Research Quarterly*, 38: 412–419.

Kurz, M.J. and Stergiou, N. (2002) 'Effect of normalisation and phase angle calculations on continuous relative phase', *Journal of Biomechanics*, 35: 369–374.

Lenth, R.V. (2001) 'Some practical guidelines for effective sample-size determination', *The American Statistician*, 55: 187–193.

Matthews, R. (1998) 'Flukes and flaws', *Prospect*, November, 20–24.

Mullineaux, D.R. and Bartlett, R.M. (1997) Research methods and statistics, in R.M. Bartlett (ed.), *Biomechanical Analysis of Movement in Sport and Exercise* (pp. 81–104), Leeds, England: British Association of Sport and Exercise Sciences.

Mullineaux, D.R. and Wheat, J. (2002) Quantifying coordination in kinematic data: a running example, in K.E. Gianikellis (ed.), *Proceedings of the 20th International Symposium on Biomechanics in Sport* (pp. 515–518), Cáceres, Spain: University of Extremadura.

Mullineaux, D.R., Barnes, C.A. and Batterham, A.M. (1999) 'Assessment of bias in comparing measurements: a reliability example', *Measurement in Physical Education and Exercise Science*, 3: 195–205.

Mullineaux, D.R., Bartlett, R.M. and Bennett, S. (2001) 'Research methods and statistics in biomechanics and motor control', *Journal of Sports Sciences*, 19: 739–760.

Mullineaux, D.R., Clayton, H.M. and Gnagey, L.M. (2004) 'Effects of offset-normalising techniques on variability in motion analysis data', *Journal of Applied Biomechanics*, 20: 177–184.

Mullineaux, D.R., Milner, C.E., Davis, I. and Hamil, J. (2006) 'Normalization of ground reaction forces', *Journal of Applied Biomechanics*, 22: 230–233.

Næs, T., Isaksson, T., Fearn, T. and Davies, T. (2002) *A User-friendly Guide to Multivariate Calibration and Classification*, Chichester, England: NIR Publications.

Park, I. and Schutz, R.W. (1999) 'Quick and easy' formulae for approximating statistical power in repeated measures ANOVA', *Measurement in Physical Education and Exercise Science*, 4: 249–270.

Peham, C., Licka, T., Girtler, D. and Scheidl, M. (2001) 'The influence of lameness on equine stride length consistency', *Veterinary Journal*, 162: 153–157.

Peters, B.T., Haddad, J.M., Heiderscheit, B.C., van Emmerik, R.E. and Hamill, J. (2003) 'Limitations in the use and interpretation of continuous relative phase', *Journal of Biomechanics*, 36: 271–274.

Pullinen, T., Mero, A., Huttunen, P., Pakarinen, A. and Komi, P V. (2002) 'Resistance exercise induced hormonal responses in men, women, and pubescent boys', *Medicine and Science in Sports and Exercise*, 34: 806–813.

Raftopoulos, D.D., Rabetas, D.A., Armstrong, C.W., Jurs, S.G. and Georgiadis, G.M. (2000) 'Evaluation of an existing and a new technique for the normalisation of ground reaction forces: total body weight versus lean body weight', *Clinical Kinesiology*, 4: 90–95.

Schmidt-Nielsen, K. (1984) *Scaling: Why is Animal Size so Important?* Cambridge: Cambridge University Press.

Shultz, B.B. and Sands, W.A. (1995) Understanding measurement concepts and statistical procedures, in P.J. Maud and C. Foster (eds), *Physiology Assessment of Human Fitness* (pp. 257–287), Champaign, IL: Human Kinetics.

Sidaway, B., Heise, G. and Schonfelder-Zohdi, B. (1995) 'Quantifying the variability of angle-angle plots', *Journal of Human Movement Studies*, 29: 181–197.

Tabachnick, B.G. and Fidell, L.S. (2001) *Using Multivariate Statistics*, Boston, MA: Allyn & Bacon.

Tanner, J.M. (1989) *Foetus into Man*, Ware, England: Castlemead.

Tepavac, D. and Field-Fote, E.C. (2001) 'Vector coding: a technique for quantification of intersegmental coupling behaviours', *Journal of Applied Biomechanics*, 17: 259–270.

Tyler, R.W. (1931) 'What is statistical significance?', *Educational Research Bulletin*, 10: 115–118.

van Weeren, P.R., van den Bogert, A.J. and Barneveld, A. (1992) 'Correction models for factors for skin displacement in equine kinematic gait analysis', *Journal of Equine Veterinary Science*, 12: 178–192.

Vincent, W.V. (1999) *Statistics in Kinesiology*, Champaign, IL: Human Kinetics.

Wheat, J.S., Bartlett, R.M., Milner, C.E. and Mullineaux, D.R. (2003) 'The effect of different surfaces on ground reaction forces during running: a single-individual design approach', *Journal of Human Movement Studies*, 44: 353–364.

Winer, B.J., Brown, D.R. and Michels, K.M. (1991) *Statistical Principles in Experimental Design*, New York, NY: McGraw-Hill.

Winter, E.M. and Nevill, A.M. (2001) Scaling: adjusting for differences in body size, in R. Eston and T. Reilly (eds), *Kinanthropometry and Exercise Physiology Laboratory Manual: Tests, Procedures and Data. Volume 1: Anthropometry* (pp. 275–293), London: Routledge.

CHAPTER 9

COMPUTER SIMULATION MODELLING IN SPORT

Maurice R. Yeadon and Mark A. King

INTRODUCTION

Experimental science aims to answer research questions by investigating the relationships between variables using quantitative data obtained in an experiment and assessing the significance of the results statistically (Yeadon and Challis, 1994). In an ideal experiment the effects of changing just one variable are determined. While it may be possible to change just one variable in a carefully controlled laboratory experiment in the natural sciences, this is problematic in the sports sciences in general and in sports biomechanics in particular. If a typical performance in a sport such as high jumping is to be investigated then any intervention must be minimal lest it make the performance atypical. For example, if the intent is to investigate the effect of run-up speed on the height reached by the mass centre in flight, asking the jumper to use various lengths of run-up might be expected to influence jumping technique minimally if the athlete normally does this in training. In such circumstances the run-up speed may be expected to vary as intended but other aspects of technique may also change. Faster approaches may be associated with a greater stride length and a more horizontal planting of the take-off leg. As a consequence the effects of a faster approach may be confounded by the effects of larger plant angles and changes in other technique variables. To isolate the relationship between approach speed and jump height statistical methods of analysis that remove the effects of other variables are needed (e.g. Greig and Yeadon, 2000). For this to be successful there must be a sufficient quantity and range of data to cope with the effects of several variables.

Theoretical approaches to answering a research question typically use a model that gives a simplified representation of the physical system under study. The main advantage of such a model is that ideal experiments can be carried out since it is possible to change just one variable. This chapter will describe theoretical models used in sports biomechanics, detailing their various components and discussing their strengths and weaknesses.

Models may be used to address the forward dynamics problem and the inverse dynamics problem. In the forward dynamics problem the driving forces are specified and the problem is to determine the resulting motion. In the inverse dynamics problem the motion is specified and the problem is to determine the driving forces that produced the motion (Zatsiorsky, 2002). Both of these types of problem will be addressed using various modelling approaches and their relative advantages will be discussed.

This chapter will first describe the process of building a mathematical model using rigid bodies and elastic structures to represent body segments and various ways of representing the force generating capabilities of muscle. Direct and indirect methods of determining the physical parameters associated with these elements will be described. Before using a model to answer a research question it is first necessary to establish that the model is an adequate representation of the real physical system. This process of model evaluation by comparing model output with real data will be discussed. Examples of applications of computer modelling will be given along with guidelines on conducting a study and reporting it.

THE FORWARD DYNAMICS PROBLEM

In the forward dynamics problem, the driving forces are specified and the problem is to determine the resulting motion. Muscle forces or joint torques may be used as the drivers in which case the joint angle time histories will be part of the resulting motion. If joint angle time histories are used as drivers for the model then the resulting motion will be specified by the whole body mass centre movement and whole body orientation time history. When a model is used in this way it is known as a simulation model.

Model building

The human body is very complex with over 200 bones and 500 muscles and, therefore, any human body model will be a simplification of reality. The degree of simplification of a simulation model will depend on the activity being simulated and the purpose of the study. For example a one-segment model of the human body may adequately represent the aerial phase of a straight dive but a model with two or three segments would be required for a piked dive to give an adequate representation. As a consequence a single model cannot be used to simulate all activities and so specific simulation models are built for particular tasks. As a general rule the model should be as simple as possible, while being sufficiently complex to address the questions set. This simple rule of thumb can be quite difficult to implement since the level of complexity needed is not always obvious.

Essentially forward dynamics simulation models can either be angle-driven, where the joint angle-time histories are input to the model and the resulting whole body orientation and mass centre position are calculated along with the required joint torques, or torque/force driven, where the joint torque- or muscle force-time histories are input to the model and the resulting kinematics are calculated. Angle-driven simulation models have typically been used to simulate activities that are not limited by strength, such as the aerial phase of sports movements including diving (Miller, 1971), high jumping (Dapena, 1981), trampolining (Yeadon et al., 1990). They have also been used in other activities, such as high bar circling (Yeadon and Hiley, 2000) or long swings on rings (Brewin et al., 2000), by limiting the joint torques to avoid unrealistic movements. Most force- or torque-driven simulation models have been used to represent relatively simple planar jumping movements, in which the human body can be represented using simplified planar two-dimensional models. In addition, movements where the body remains symmetrical about the sagittal plane, such as swinging on rings (Sprigings et al., 1998), have often been modelled as this allows the simulation model to have fewer segments and hence fewer degrees of freedom.

Angle-driven models have typically been more complex with more segments and degrees of freedom as they are easier to control while torque-driven models have been relatively simple in general, owing to the difficulties in determining realistic parameters for muscles. One notable exception is the jumping model of Hatze, 1981a, which simulated the take-off phase in long jumping. This model comprised 17 segments and 46 muscle groups but did not simulate the impact phase and did not allow for soft tissue movement.

Model components

The following section will discuss the various components that are used to build a typical simulation model.

Linked segment models

Most of the whole body simulation models in sports biomechanics are based on a collection of rigid bodies (segments) linked together, and are generically called 'linked segment systems'. The rigid bodies are the principal building blocks of simulation models and can be thought of as representing the basic structure and inertia of the human body. For each rigid segment in a planar model four parameters are usually required: length, mass, mass centre location, and moment of inertia. The number of segments used depends on the aim of the study and the activity being modelled. For example, Alexander, 1990, used a two-segment model to determine optimum approach speeds in jumps for height and distance, Neptune and Kautz, 2000, used a planar two-legged bicycle-rider model to look at muscle contributions in forward and backward pedalling, and King and Yeadon, 2003, used a planar five-segment model to investigate take-offs in tumbling. The complexity needed is not always obvious.

Torque-free two-segment models of vaulting have been used to show that the backward rotation generated during the take-off of a Hecht vault is largely a function of the velocity and configuration at initial contact together with the passive mechanics during impact (Sprigings and Yeadon, 1997; King et al., 1999). These results were confirmed using a torque-driven five-segment model but it was also shown that the inclusion of a hand segment and shoulder elasticity made substantial contributions to rotation (King and Yeadon, 2005).

Wobbling masses

Although linked rigid body models have been used extensively to model many activities, a recent development has been to modify some of the rigid segments in the model by incorporating wobbling mass elements (Gruber et al., 1998). This type of representation allows some of the mass (soft tissue) in a segment to move relative to the bone, the rigid part. For impacts the inclusion of wobbling masses within the model is crucial as the loading on the system can be up to nearly 50 per cent lower for a wobbling mass model compared with the equivalent rigid segment model (Pain and Challis, 2006). The most common way to model wobbling masses is to attach a second rigid element to the first fixed rigid element, representing the bone, within a segment using non-linear damped passive springs with spring force $F = kx^3 - d\dot{x}$ where x is displacement, $\dot{x}$ is velocity and k and d are constants (Pain and Challis, 2001a).

The disadvantage of including wobbling mass elements within a simulation model is that there are more parameter values to determine and the equations of motion are more complex leading to longer simulation times. Wobbling mass segments should, therefore, only be included when necessary. Whether to include wobbling masses depends on the activity being modelled, although it is not always obvious whether they are needed. For example a simulation model of springboard diving (Yeadon et al., 2006b) included wobbling mass segments, but when the springs were made 500 times stiffer the resulting simulations were almost identical.

Connection between rigid links

Typically the rigid links in the simulation model are joined together by frictionless joints, whereby adjacent segments share a common line or a common point. For example Neptune and Kautz, 2000, used a hinge joint to allow for flexion–extension at the knee while Hatze, 1981a, used a universal joint at the hip with three degrees of freedom to allow for flexion–extension, abduction–adduction and internal–external rotation. The assumption that adjacent segments share a common point or line is a simplification of reality and, although reasonable for most joints, it is questionable at the shoulder where motion occurs at four different joints. Models of the shoulder joint have ranged in complexity from a one degree of freedom pin joint (Yeadon and King, 2002) to relatively simple viscoelastic representations (Hiley and

Yeadon, 2003a) and complex finite element models (van der Helm, 1994). The complexity to be used depends on the requirements of the study. Simple viscoelastic representations have been used successfully in whole body models where the overall movement is of interest whereas complex models have been used to address issues such as the contribution of individual muscles to movement at the shoulder joint.

Interface with external surface

The simplest way to model contact between a human body model and an external surface, such as the ground or sports equipment, is to use a 'joint' so that the model rotates about a fixed point on the external surface (Bobbert et al., 2002). The disadvantage of this method is that it does not allow the model to translate relative to the point of contact or allow for a collision with the external surface since for an impact to occur the velocity of the point contacting the surface has to be non-zero initially. Alternatively forces can be applied at a finite number of locations using viscoelastic elements at the interface with the forces determined by the displacements and velocities of the points in contact. The viscoelastic elements can be used to represent specific elastic structures within the body such as the heel pad (Pain and Challis, 2001b) or sports equipment such as the high bar (Hiley and Yeadon, 2003b) or tumble track-foot interface (King and Yeadon, 2004). The equations used for the viscoelastic elements have varied in complexity from simple damped linear representations (King and Yeadon, 2004) through to highly non-linear equations (Wright et al., 1998). The number of points of contact varies but it is typically less than three (Yeadon and King, 2002) although 66 points of contact were used to simulate heel–toe running (Wright et al., 1998). The horizontal forces acting while in contact with an external surface can be calculated using a friction model (Gerritsen et al., 1995) where the horizontal force is expressed as a function of the vertical force and the horizontal velocity of the point in contact or by using viscoelastic springs (Yeadon and King, 2002). If viscoelastic springs are used the horizontal force should be expressed as a function of the vertical force so that the horizontal force falls to zero at the same time as the vertical force (Wilson et al., 2006).

Muscle models

Muscle models in sports biomechanics are typically based upon the work of A.V. Hill where the force-producing capabilities of muscle are divided into contractile and elastic elements (lumped parameter models) with the most commonly used version being the three-component Hill model (Caldwell, 2004). The model consists of a contractile element and two elastic elements, the series elastic element and the parallel elastic element. Mathematical relationships are required for each element in the muscle model so that the force exerted by a muscle on the simulation model can be defined throughout a simulation.

Contractile element

The force that a contractile element produces can be expressed as a function of three factors; muscle length, muscle velocity and muscle activation. The force–length relationship for a muscle is well documented as being bell-shaped with small tensions at extremes of length and maximal tension in between (Edman, 1992). As a consequence, the force–length relationship is often modelled as a simple quadratic function.

The force–velocity relationship for a muscle can be split into two parts, the concentric phase and the eccentric phase. In the concentric phase tetanic muscle force decreases hyperbolically with increasing speed of shortening to approach zero at maximum shortening speed (Hill, 1938). In the eccentric phase maximum tetanic muscle force increases rapidly to around 1.4–1.5 times the isometric value with increasing speed of lengthening and then plateaus for higher speeds (Dudley *et al.*, 1990; Harry *et al.*, 1990). Maximum voluntary muscle force shows a similar force–velocity relationship in the concentric phase, but plateaus at 1.1–1.2 times the isometric value in the eccentric phase (Westing *et al.*, 1988; Yeadon, King and Wilson, 2006a).

The voluntary activation level of a muscle ranges from 0 (no activation) to 1 (maximum voluntary activation) during a simulation and is defined as a function of time. This function is multiplied by the maximum voluntary force given by the force–length and force–velocity relationships to give the muscle force exerted. Ideally the function used to define the activation time history of a muscle should have only a few parameters. One way of doing this is to define a simple activation profile for each muscle (basic shape) using a few parameters (Yeadon and King, 2002). For example, in jumping, the activations of the extensors rise up from a low initial value to a maximum and then drop off towards the end of the simulation, while the flexor activations drop from an initial to a low value and then rise towards the end of the simulation (King, Wilson and Yeadon, 2006). These parameters are varied within realistic limits to define the activation-time history used for each muscle during a specific simulation.

Series elastic element

The series elastic element represents the connective tissue – the tendon and aponeurosis – in series with the contractile element. The force produced by the series elastic element is typically expressed as an increasing function of its length with a slack length below which no force can be generated. It is usually assumed that the series elastic element stretches by around five per cent at maximum isometric force (Muramatsu *et al.*, 2001).

Parallel elastic element

The effect of the parallel elastic element is often ignored in models of sports movements as this element does not produce high forces for the normal working ranges of joints (Chapman, 1985).

Torque generators vs. individual muscle representations

All simulation models that include individual muscle models have the disadvantage that it is very difficult to determine individual parameters for each element of each muscle, as it is impossible to measure all the parameters required non-invasively. As a consequence, researchers rely on data from the literature for their muscle models and so the models are not specific to an individual. An alternative approach is to use torque generators to represent the net effect of all the muscles crossing a joint (e.g. King and Yeadon, 2002) as the net torque produced by a group of muscles can be measured on a constant velocity dynamometer. More recently the extensor and flexor muscle groups around a joint have been represented by separate torque generators (King *et al.*, 2006). In both cases each torque generator consists of rotational elastic and contractile elements. Using torque generators instead of individual muscles gives similar mathematical relationships with the maximum voluntary torque produced by the contractile element being expressed as a function of the muscle angle and muscle angular velocity (Yeadon *et al.*, 2006a).

Model construction

The following sections will discuss the process of building a simulation model and running simulations using the components described in the previous section.

Free body diagram of the model

A free-body diagram of a simulation model gives all the necessary information required to build the computer simulation model. The free-body diagram should include the segments, the forces and torques and the nomenclature for lengths (Figure 9.1). In the system shown there are two degrees of freedom since the two angles θ_a and θ_b define the orientation and configuration of the model.

Generating the equations of motion

The equations of motion for a mechanical system can be generated from first principles using Newton's Second Law for relatively simple models with only a few segments (e.g. Hiley and Yeadon, 2003b). For a planar link model, three equations of motion are available for each segment using Newton's Second Law (force, F, = mass × acceleration, m a) in two perpendicular directions and taking moments (moment, T, = moment of inertia × angular acceleration, I α) for each segment. In Figure 9.1 this allows the calculation of one angle and two reaction forces for each segment.

   For more complex models a computer package is recommended, as it can take a long time to generate the equations of motion by hand and the likelihood of making errors is high. There are several commercially available

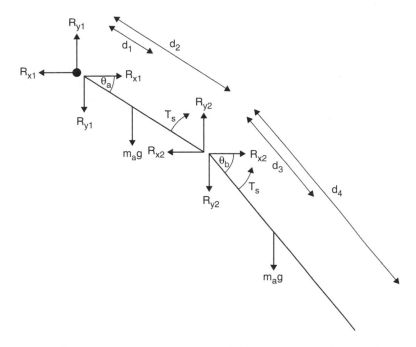

Figure 9.1   Free body diagram of a two-segment model of a gymnast swinging around a high bar

software packages, for example DADS, ADAMS, AUTOLEV and SD Fast, that can generate equations of motion for a user-defined system of rigid and elastic elements. Each package allows the user to input a relatively simple description of the model and the equations of motion are then automatically generated, solved and integrated. Note that with all packages that automatically generate equations of motion, it is important to learn how to use the specific software by building simple models and performing checks to ensure that the results are correct. Some packages, such as AUTOLEV, generate computer source code, typically FORTRAN or C, for the mechanical system. The advantage of this is that the user can then customise the basic simulation model to incorporate muscle models or an optimisation routine, for example. Other more complex packages do not give full access to the source code and this can prevent the model from being customised for specific tasks.

Model input and output

Two sets of input are required for a simulation to run. First, there are the initial kinematics, which comprises the mass centre velocity, and the orientation and angular velocity of each segment. The initial kinematics can be obtained from recordings of actual performances, although it can be difficult to obtain accurate velocity estimates (Hubbard and Alaways, 1989). Secondly, there is information required during the simulation. A kinematically driven model requires joint angle-time histories (Yeadon, 1990a) while a kinetically driven model requires activation histories for each actuator (muscle or torque generator) in the model (Alexander, 1990; Neptune and Hull, 1999).

The output from both types of simulation model comprises time histories of all the variables calculated in the simulation model. For a kinematically driven model this is the whole-body orientation, linear and angular momentum and joint torques, while for a kinetically driven model it comprises the whole-body orientation, linear and angular momentum and joint angle-time histories.

Integration

Running a simulation to calculate how a model moves, requires a method for integrating the equations of motion over time. The simplest method to increment a set of equations of motion (ordinary differential equations) through a time interval dt is to use derivative information from the beginning of the interval. This is known as the 'Euler method' (Press *et al.*, 1988):

$$x_{n+1} = x_x + \dot{x}_n dt + \tfrac{1}{2}\ddot{x}_n dt^2$$

where x, $\dot{x}$, $\ddot{x}$ are, respectively, the displacement, velocity and acceleration and suffices n and $n + 1$ denote the nth and $(n + 1)$ step separated by a step length dt. The Euler method assumes a fixed step length of dt, where dt is equal to 0.0001 s, for example. The disadvantage of the Euler method is that a comparatively small step size is needed and the method is not very stable (Press *et al.*, 1988). A better method is to use a fourth order Runge–Kutta in which four evaluations of the function are calculated per step size (Press *et al.*, 1988). In addition, most good integration routines include a variable step size with the aim to have some predetermined accuracy in a solution with minimum computational effort (Press *et al.*, 1988).

A kinetically driven model requires the force or torque produced by each actuator to be input to the model at each time step. The force or torque produced is a function of the actuator's activation, length and velocity. The movement of the contractile element or series elastic element must, therefore, be calculated. Caldwell, 2004, gives an in-depth account of this procedure, but essentially at each time step the total length of the actuator is split between the contractile element and series elastic element in such a way that the force or torque in each element are equal.

Error checking

Whatever method is used to generate the equations of motion, it is always important that checks are carried out to ensure that no simple programming errors have been made. Examples are: energy is conserved if all damping is removed and all the muscles are switched off; the mass centre of the model follows a parabola if the forces between the simulation model and the external surface are set to zero; impulse equals change in linear momentum; angular momentum about the mass centre is conserved during flight.

Optimisation

Simulation models can be used to find the optimum technique for a specific task by running many simulations with different inputs. To perform an optimisation is a three stage process. Firstly, an objective function, or performance score, must be formulated which can be maximised or minimised by varying inputs to the model within realistic limits. For jumping simulations the objective function can simply be the jump height or jump distance, but for movements in which rotation is also important a more complex function incorporating both mass centre movement and rotation is required. The challenge for formulating such an objective function is to determine appropriate weightings for each variable in the function since the weightings affect the solution.

Secondly, realistic limits need to be established for each of the variables, typically activation parameters to each muscle and initial conditions. Additionally the activation patterns of each muscle need to be defined using only a few parameters to keep the optimisation run time reasonably low and increase the likelihood of finding a global optimum.

Thirdly, an algorithm capable of finding the global optimum rather than a local optimum is needed. Of the many algorithms available the Simplex algorithm (Nelder and Mead, 1965), the Simulated Annealing algorithm (Goffe et al., 1994) and Genetic algorithms (van Soest and Cassius, 2003) have proved popular. The Simplex algorithm typically finds a solution quickly but can get stuck at a local optimum as it only accepts downhill solutions, whereas the Simulated Annealing and Genetic algorithms are better at finding the global optimum as they can escape from local optima.

Summary of model construction

- Decide which factors are important.
- Decide upon the number of segments and joints.
- Decide whether to include wobbling masses.
- Draw the free body diagram showing all the forces acting on the system.
- Decide whether the model is to be angle-driven or torque-driven.
- Decide which muscles should be represented.
- Decide how to model the interface with the ground or equipment.
- Decide whether to use a software package or to build the model from first principles.

Parameter determination

Determining parameters for a simulation model is difficult but vital, as the values chosen can have a large influence on the resulting simulations. Parameters are needed for the rigid and wobbling mass segments, muscle–tendon complexes, and viscoelastic elements in the model. Fundamentally there are two different ways to approach this, either to estimate values from the literature, or take measurements on an individual to determine individual-specific parameters. There is a clear advantage to determining individual-specific parameters as it allows a model to be evaluated by comparing simulation output with performance data on the same individual.

Inertia parameters

Accurate segmental inertia values are needed for each segment in the simulation model. For a rigid segment the inertia parameters consist of the segmental mass, length, mass centre location and moment of inertia; one moment of inertia value is needed for a planar model, while three moment of inertia values are needed for a three-dimensional model. For a wobbling mass segment there are twice as many inertia parameters needed since a wobbling mass segment comprises two rigid bodies connected by viscoelastic springs.

There are two methods of obtaining rigid segmental inertia parameters. The first is to use regression equations (Hinrichs, 1985; Yeadon and Morlock, 1989) based upon anthropometric measurements and inertia parameters determined from cadaver segments (Dempster, 1955; Chandler, 1975). The disadvantage of this method is that the accuracy is dependent on how well the morphology of the participant compares with the cadavers used in the study. A better method, which only requires density values from cadaver studies, is to take anthropometric measurements on the participant and use a geometric model (Jensen, 1978; Hatze, 1980; Yeadon, 1990b) to determine the segmental inertia parameters. Although it is difficult to establish the accuracy of these geometric models for determining segmental inertia parameters, error values of around two per cent have been reported for total body mass (Yeadon, 1990b).

An alternative method that is worthy of mention is to use medical imaging techniques (Martin *et al.*, 1989; Zatsiorsky *et al.*, 1990) to determine segmental inertia parameters. With current technology and ethical issues this approach is not a real alternative at present but in the future it might provide a means for determining individual-specific segmental density values or provide a means for evaluating other methods for determining individual-specific segmental inertia parameters.

Including wobbling mass segments within the model increases the number of unknown parameters that are needed for each segment. The combined segmental inertia parameters can be calculated using a geometric model or regression equations. However, the calculation of the inertia parameters of the separate fixed and wobbling masses requires additional information on the ratio of bone to soft tissue, which is typically obtained from cadaver dissection studies (Clarys and Marfell-Jones, 1986). These ratio data can then be scaled to the specific individual using total body mass and percentage body fat (Pain and Challis, 2006; Wilson *et al.*, 2006). In the future it may be possible to improve this method by determining the inertia parameters for the rigid and wobbling masses of each segment directly from medical imaging.

Strength parameters

Determining accurate individual-specific strength parameters for muscle–tendon complexes is a major challenge in sports biomechanics, which has resulted in two different ways to represent the forces produced by muscles. The first is to include all the major muscles that cross a joint in the simulation model as individual muscle–tendon complexes with the parameters for the individual muscles obtained mainly from animal experiments (e.g. Gerritsen *et al.*, 1995). Although the parameters are sometimes scaled to an individual or group of individuals based upon isometric measurements (Hatze, 1981b) this method does not give a complete set of individual-specific strength parameters. The alternative approach is to use torque generators at each joint in the model to represent the effect of all the muscles around a joint (flexors and extensors represented by separate torque generators). The advantage of this approach is that the net torque at a given joint can be measured on a constant velocity dynamometer over a range of joint angular velocities and joint angles for the participant and so individual-specific parameters can be determined that define maximal voluntary torque as a function of muscle angle and velocity (King and Yeadon, 2002; Yeadon *et al.*, 2006a). With this approach it is still necessary to use data from the literature to determine the parameters for the series elastic element for each torque generator. In recent studies (King *et al.*, 2006) it has been assumed that the series elastic element stretches by 5 per cent of its resting length during isometric contractions (De Zee and Voigt, 2001; Muramatsu *et al.*, 2001). Although it would be desirable to be able to determine series elastic element parameters directly from measurements on an individual, it has previously been shown that simulation results were not sensitive to these parameter values (Yeadon and King, 2002).

Viscoelastic parameters

Viscoelastic parameters are required for springs that are included within a simulation model: connection of wobbling masses, shoulder joint, foot– or hand–ground interface and equipment. Sometimes these springs represent specific elements where it is possible to determine viscoelastic properties from measurements (Pain and Challis, 2001b) while in other models the springs represent more than one viscoelastic element and so make it much harder to determine the parameters from experiments (e.g. Yeadon and King, 2002). Viscoelastic parameters should ideally be determined from independent tests and then fixed within the model for all simulations (Gerritsen *et al.*, 1995; Pain and Challis, 2001a). If this is not possible the viscoelastic parameters can be determined through an optimisation procedure by choosing initial values and then allowing the parameters to vary within realistic bounds until an optimum match between simulation and performance is found. With this method a torque-driven or angle-driven simulation model can be used, although it is easier to implement in an angle-driven model as the joint angle changes are specified and so there are less parameters to be determined. Optimising the parameter values has the potential for the springs to compensate for errors in the model.

This can be overcome by using a small set of spring parameters, determining the parameters from more than one trial and then fixing the parameter values for the model evaluation. For example Yeadon and King, 2002, determined viscoelastic parameters for the interface between foot and tumble track from one trial using a torque-driven model and then evaluated the model on a different trial, while Yeadon et al., 2006b, determined viscoelastic parameters for the interface of a diver with a springboard from four trials using an angle-driven model. Using more than one trial for determining the spring parameters also has the advantage that the model output should not be overly sensitive to the parameter values used.

Model evaluation

Model evaluation is an essential step in the process of developing a simulation model and should be carried out before a model is used in applications. Although this step was identified as an important part of the process over 25 years ago (Panjabi, 1979) the weakness of many simulation models is still that their accuracy is unknown (Yeadon and Challis, 1994). While a number of models have been evaluated to some extent, such as those of Hatze, 1981a; Yeadon et al., 1990; Neptune and Hull, 1998; Brewin et al., 2000; Fujii and Hubbard, 2002; Yeadon and King, 2002; Hiley and Yeadon, 2003a; and King et al., 2006, many have not been evaluated at all.

The complexity of the model and its intended use should be taken into account when evaluating a model. For a simple model (e.g. Alexander, 1990), which is used to make general predictions, it may be sufficient to show that results are of the correct magnitude. In contrast, if a model is being used to investigate the factors that determine optimum performance in jumping, the model should be evaluated quantitatively so that the accuracy of the model is known (e.g. King et al., 2006). Ideally the model evaluation should encompass the range of initial conditions and activities that the model is used for with little extrapolation of the model to cases in which the accuracy is unknown (Panjabi, 1979). For example, if a simulation model of springboard diving is evaluated successfully for forward dives, the model may not work for reverse dives and so it should be also evaluated using reverse dives.

The purpose of model evaluation is to determine the accuracy, which can then be borne in mind when considering the results of simulations. Furthermore a successful evaluation gives confidence that the model assumptions are not erroneous and that there are no gross modelling defects or simulation software errors. Ideally the evaluation process should include all aspects of the model that are going to be used to make predictions. If a model is going to be used to investigate the effect of initial conditions on maximum jump height then the model should be evaluated quantitatively to show that for a given set of initial conditions the model can perform the movement in a similar way and produce a similar jump height. If a model is to be used to examine how the knee flexor and extensor muscles are used in jumping, the model should be evaluated to show that for a given jump the model uses similar muscle forces to the actual performance.

To evaluate a simulation model is challenging and may require several iterations of model development before the model is evaluated satisfactorily. Initially data must be collected on an actual performance by the sports participant. Ideally this should be an elite performer who is able to work maximally throughout the testing and produce a performance that is close to optimal. Time histories of kinematic variables, from video or an automatic system, kinetic variables from force plate or force transducers, and electromyograms (EMG) histories, if possible, should be obtained. Individual-specific model parameter values, such as anthropometry and strength, are then determined from the measurements taken on the individual, with as little reliance on data from the literature as possible (Wilson *et al.*, 2006; Yeadon *et al.*, 2006a). The initial kinematic conditions (positions and velocities) for the model are then determined from the performance data and input to the model along with any other time histories that are required for the model to run a single simulation. If the model is kinetically driven this will consist of the activation-time history for each actuator (Yeadon and King, 2002), while if the model is kinematically driven the time history of each joint angle will be required (Hiley and Yeadon, 2003a). Once a single simulation has been run, a difference score should be calculated by quantitatively comparing the simulation with the actual performance. The formulation of the score depends on the activity being simulated, but it should include all features of the performance that the model should match, such as joint angle changes, linear and angular momentum, and floor movement. The difficulty in combining severable variables into one score is that appropriate weightings need to be chosen for each part of the objective function. For example Yeadon and King, 2002, assumed that a 1° difference in a joint angle at take-off was equivalent to a one per cent difference in mass centre velocity at take-off. Furthermore, for variables that cannot be measured accurately, such as wobbling mass movement, it may be more appropriate to add a penalty to the difference score if too much movement occurs (King *et al.*, 2006). Finally the input to the model is then varied until the best comparison is found (score minimised) using an optimisation routine. If the comparison between performance and simulation is close (Figure 9.2) then the model can be used to run simulations. If not then the model complexity or model parameters need to be modified and the

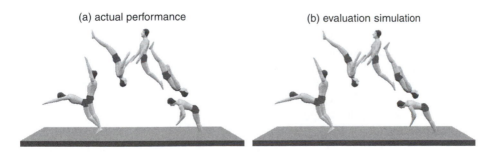

(a) actual performance   (b) evaluation simulation

Figure 9.2 Comparison of performance and simulation graphics for the tumbling model of Yeadon and King, 2002

model re-evaluated. If the comparison gives a percentage difference of less than 10 per cent this is often sufficient for applications in sports biomechanics.

Issues in model design

The design of a particular model should be driven by the intended use and the questions to be answered. For example, if the aim is to determine the forces that act within the human body during running then an inverse dynamics model may be more appropriate than a forward dynamics model. If the aim is to demonstrate some general mechanical principles for a type of movement then a simple model may be adequate. The issue of model complexity is not simple, however. While it is evident that simple models such as Alexander's (1990) model of jumping can give insight into the mechanics of technique, there is often a tendency to rely on the quantitative results without recourse to model evaluation. The issue of model evaluation for a simple model is problematic since all that can be realistically expected is a ballpark or order-of-magnitude accuracy. To achieve anything approaching 10 per cent accuracy when compared with actual performance a model of some complexity is usually required, comprising several segments, realistic joint drivers and elastic elements. The development of such a model is a non-trivial endeavour. Sprigings and Miller, 2004, argue the case for "the use of the simplest possible model capable of capturing the essence of the task being studied", citing Alexander, 1990, and Hubbard, 1993, in support. The problem here is deciding at what point a model is too simple. If a model is so simple that it is 30 per cent inaccurate then it is difficult to justify conclusions indicated by the model results unless they are robust to a 30 per cent inaccuracy. It is evident that some measure of model accuracy is needed to reach conclusions.

Simple models of throwing in which the implement is modelled as an aerodynamic rigid body (Hubbard and Alaways, 1987) need to be complemented by a representation of the ability of the thrower to impart velocity in a given direction (Hubbard et al., 2001) so that realistic simulations may be carried out. The same considerations apply to other models that do not include the human participant.

While a rigid body may be adequate for a model of equipment it is likely to be too simple for a model of an activity such as high jumping (Hubbard and Trinkle, 1985a; b) although a rigid body model has been used to give insight into the two general modes of rotational aerial motion (Yeadon, 1993a).

Joint angle time histories are sometimes used as drivers for a simulation model. In the case of aerial movement (van Gheluwe, 1981; Yeadon et al., 1990) it can be argued that this is a reasonable approach so long as the angular velocities are limited to achievable values. In activities where there are large contact forces with the external surroundings this approach is more problematic since steps need to be taken to ensure that the corresponding joint torques are achievable. Hiley and Yeadon, 2003a; b and Brewin et al., 2000, used angle-driven models to simulate swinging on the high bar and on the rings and eliminated simulations that required larger torques than were achieved by the participant on a constant velocity dynamometer. Another approach is to use joint torques as drivers where the maximum voluntary joint torque is a function of angular velocity (Alexander, 1990) and, possibly, of joint angle (King and Yeadon, 2003). This approach leads to more realistic simulations than the use of angle-driven models but there is a corresponding loss of the simple control of joint angles. Finally there are models that use representations of individual muscles or muscle groups crossing a joint (Hatze, 1981a; Neptune and Hull, 1998) and these have the potential to provide even more accurate representations but pose the problem of determining appropriate muscle parameter values.

Reviews of computer simulation modelling are provided by Miller, 1975; King, 1984; Vaughan, 1984; Yeadon, 1987; Vaughan, 1989; Hubbard, 1993; and Alexander, 2003.

THE INVERSE DYNAMICS PROBLEM

The inverse dynamics problem is to determine the forces that must act to produce a given motion. Theoretically the only information needed comprises the time histories of the variables that define the motion of the system. From a practical perspective, however, estimates of angular accelerations from the given data typically have large errors and so additional information is often provided in the form of recorded ground reaction forces. As an example a four-segment model representing a handstand on a force plate will be used to determine the torques acting at each joint.

An inverse dynamics model of a handstand

The body is represented by four rigid segments H, A, B, C representing the hands, arms, trunk+head, and legs (Figures 9.3 and 9.4). Newton–Euler equations are used to generate three equations per segment for the six joint reaction forces, three angular accelerations and three joint torques. This system of 12 equations in 12 unknowns is reduced to a system of six equations in the joint accelerations and joint torques by eliminating the six reaction forces. A knowledge of the segmental inertia parameters of a gymnast together with the time histories of the three joint angles during a handstand then permits the calculation of the joint torque time histories.

Each of the four segments in Figure 9.3 {Hand (H), Figure 9.3a; Arm (A), Figure 9.3b; Body, (B), Figure 9.3c; Leg (C), Figure 9.3d} produces three equations: one for resultant vertical force, one for resultant horizontal force, one for moments about the mass centre.

For Figure 9.3a:

$$\uparrow : R - R_1 - m_h g = 0 \tag{9.1}$$

$$\rightarrow : F - F_1 = 0 \tag{9.2}$$

$$H : -T_1 + R(x_p - x_h) + R_1(x_h - x_1) + F(z_h - z_p) + F_1(z_1 - z_h) = 0 \tag{9.3}$$

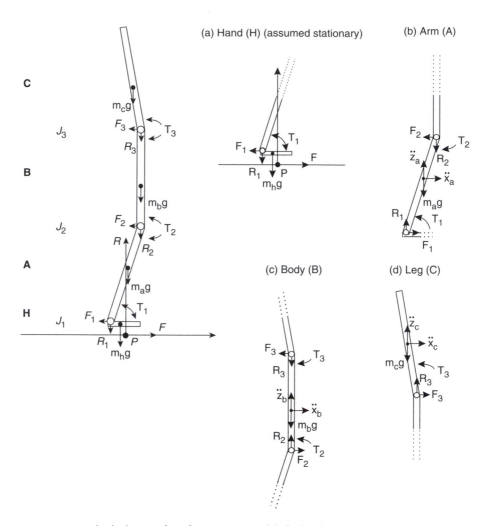

Figure 9.3 Free body diagram for a four-segment model of a handstand

H	: hand segment
A	: arm segment
B	: body (trunk and head) segment
C	: leg segment
J_1	: wrist joint
J_2	: shoulder joint
J_3	: hip joint
(x_i, z_i)	: joint centre coordinates $(i = 1, 3)$
F_i	: horizontal joint reaction forces $(i = 1, 3)$
R_i	: vertical joint reaction forces $(i = 1, 3)$
T_j	: torque about joint centre J_i $(i = 1, 3)$
P	: centre of pressure
F	: horizontal reaction force on H
R	: vertical reaction force on H
(x_j, z_j)	: segment mass centre coordinates $(j = h, a, b$ or c)
(x_p, z_p)	: point of force application $(z_p$ is assumed $= 0)$
$\ddot{x}_j$	: horizontal linear accelerations of segment mass centre $(j = h, a, b$ or c)
$\ddot{z}_j$	: vertical linear accelerations of segment mass centres $(j = h, a, b$ or c)
m_j	: segment mass $(j = h, a, b$ or c)
I_j	: moment of inertia about segment mass centres $(j = h, a, b$ or c)
$\ddot{\phi}_j$	: segment angular accelerations $(j = h, a, b$ or c)
g	: acceleration due to gravity

For Figure 9.3b:

$$\uparrow : R_1 - R_2 - m_ag = m_a\ddot{z}_a \tag{9.4}$$

$$\rightarrow : F_1 - F_2 = m_a\ddot{x}_a \tag{9.5}$$

$$A : -T_2 + T_1 + F_1(z_a - z_1) + F_2(z_2 - z_a) - R_1(x_a - x_1)$$
$$- R_2(x_2 - x_a) = I_a\ddot{\phi}_a \tag{9.6}$$

For Figure 9.3c:

$$\uparrow : R_2 - R_3 - m_bg = m_b\ddot{z}_b \tag{9.7}$$

$$\rightarrow : F_2 - F_3 = m_b\ddot{x}_b \tag{9.8}$$

$$B : T_2 - T_3 + F_2(z_b - z_2) + F_3(z_3 - z_b) - R_2(x_b - x_2)$$
$$- R_3(x_3 - x_b) = I_b\ddot{\phi}_b \tag{9.9}$$

For Figure 9.3d:

$$\uparrow : R_3 - m_cg = m_c\ddot{z}_c \tag{9.10}$$

$$\rightarrow : F_3 = m_c\ddot{x}_c \tag{9.11}$$

$$C : T_3 + F_3(z_c - z_3) - R_3(x_c - x_3) = I_c\ddot{\phi}_c \tag{9.12}$$

Combining equations $(9.1) + (9.4) + (9.7) + (9.10)$ resolves forces vertically for the whole system to give:

$$R - mg = m_a\ddot{z}_a + m_b\ddot{z}_b + m_c\ddot{z}_c \tag{9.13}$$

Combining equations $(9.2) + (9.5) + (9.8) + (9.11)$ resolves forces horizontally for the whole system to give:

$$F = m_a\ddot{x}_a + m_b\ddot{x}_b + m_c\ddot{x}_c \tag{9.14}$$

Substituting for values R_1 and F_1 in (9.3) is equivalent to taking moments about J_1 for H and gives:

$$T_1 = F(z_1 - z_p) + R(x_p - x_1) - m_hg(x_h - x_1) \tag{9.15}$$

Combining equations (9.15) and (9.6), substituting for R_2 and F_2 is equivalent to taking moments about J_2 for H and A and gives:

$$F(z_2 - z_p) - R(x_2 - x_p) + m_hg(x_2 - x_h) + m_ag(x_2 - x_a)$$
$$= T_2 + I_a\ddot{\phi}_a + m_a\ddot{x}_a(z_2 - z_a) - m_a\ddot{z}_a(x_2 - x_a) \tag{9.16}$$

Combining equations (9.16) and (9.9), substituting for R_3 and F_3 and taking moments about J_3 for H, A and B gives:

$$F(z_3 - z_p) - R(x_3 - x_p) + m_hg(x_3 - x_h) + m_ag(x_3 - x_a) + m_bg(x_3 - x_b)$$
$$= T_3 + I_a\ddot{\phi}_a + I_b\ddot{\phi}_b + m_a\ddot{x}_a(z_3 - z_a) + m_a\ddot{x}_b(z_3 - z_b)$$
$$- m_a\ddot{z}_a(x_3 - x_a) - m_b\ddot{z}_b(x_3 - x_b) \tag{9.17}$$

Combining equations (9.17) and (9.12) is equivalent to taking moments about P for the whole system and gives:

$$-mg(x - x_p) = I_a\ddot{\phi}_a + I_b\ddot{\phi}_b + I_c\ddot{\phi}_c - m_a\ddot{x}_a(z_a - z_p) - m_b\ddot{x}_b(z_b - z_p)$$
$$- m_c\ddot{x}_c(z_c - z_p) + m_a\ddot{z}_a(x_a - x_p) + m_b\ddot{z}_b(x_b - x_p)$$
$$+ m_c\ddot{z}_c(x_c - x_p) \tag{9.18}$$

Therefore, eliminating reactions at joints has left six equations of motion. Using the representation of Figure 9.4, the geometric equivalents of segment mass centre linear accelerations can be obtained by differentiating the position values twice.

$$x_a = x_1 + a_1 \cos \phi_a$$
$$\ddot{x}_a = -a_1 \sin \phi_a \ddot{\phi}_a - a_1 \cos \phi_a \dot{\phi}_a^2$$

$$z_a = z_1 + a_1 \sin \phi_a$$
$$\ddot{z}_a = -a_1 \cos \phi_a \ddot{\phi}_a - a_1 \sin \phi_a \dot{\phi}_a^2$$

$$x_b = x_1 + a_2 \cos \phi_a + b_1 \cos \phi_b$$
$$\ddot{x}_b = -a_2 \sin \phi_a \ddot{\phi}_a - a_2 \cos \phi_a \dot{\phi}_a^2 - b_1 \sin \phi_b \ddot{\phi}_b - b_1 \cos \phi_b \dot{\phi}_b^2$$

$$z_b = z_1 + a_2 \sin \phi_a + b_1 \sin \phi_b$$
$$\ddot{z}_b = a_2 \cos \phi_a \ddot{\phi}_a - a_2 \sin \phi_a \dot{\phi}_a^2 + b_1 \cos \phi_b \ddot{\phi}_b - b_1 \sin \phi_b \dot{\phi}_b^2$$

$$x_c = x_1 + a_2 \cos \phi_a + b_2 \cos \phi_b + c_1 \cos \phi_c$$
$$\ddot{x}_c = -a_2 \sin \phi_a \ddot{\phi}_a - a_2 \cos \phi_a \dot{\phi}_a^2 - b_2 \sin \phi_b \ddot{\phi}_b - b_2 \cos \phi_b \dot{\phi}_b^2 - c_1 \sin \phi_c \ddot{\phi}_c - c_1 \cos \phi_c \dot{\phi}_c^2$$

$$z_c = z_1 + a_2 \sin \phi_a + b_2 \sin \phi_b + c_1 \sin \phi_c$$
$$\ddot{z}_c = a_2 \cos \phi_a \ddot{\phi}_a - a_2 \sin \phi_a \dot{\phi}_a^2 + b_2 \cos \phi_b \ddot{\phi}_b - b_2 \sin \phi_b \dot{\phi}_b^2 + c_1 \cos \phi_c \ddot{\phi}_c - c_1 \sin \phi_c \dot{\phi}_c^2$$

By substituting the geometric equivalents in place of the linear acceleration terms in equations (9.13)–(9.18) and re-arranging terms, we obtain

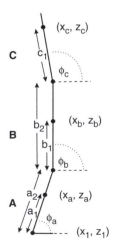

Figure 9.4 Four-segment model of a handstand

six linear equations in the following form to solve for six unknowns $(T_1, T_2, T_3, \phi_a, \phi_b, \phi_c)$.

$$A_{11}T_1 + A_{12}T_2 + A_{13}T_3 + A_{14}\ddot{\phi}_a + A_{15}\ddot{\phi}_b + A_{16}\ddot{\phi}_c = B_1$$
$$A_{21}T_1 + A_{22}T_2 + A_{23}T_3 + A_{24}\ddot{\phi}_a + A_{25}\ddot{\phi}_b + A_{26}\ddot{\phi}_c = B_2$$
$$A_{31}T_1 + A_{32}T_2 + A_{33}T_3 + A_{34}\ddot{\phi}_a + A_{35}\ddot{\phi}_b + A_{36}\ddot{\phi}_c = B_3$$
$$A_{41}T_1 + A_{42}T_2 + A_{43}T_3 + A_{44}\ddot{\phi}_a + A_{45}\ddot{\phi}_b + A_{46}\ddot{\phi}_c = B_4$$
$$A_{51}T_1 + A_{52}T_2 + A_{53}T_3 + A_{54}\ddot{\phi}_a + A_{55}\ddot{\phi}_b + A_{56}\ddot{\phi}_c = B_5$$
$$A_{61}T_1 + A_{62}T_2 + A_{63}T_3 + A_{64}\ddot{\phi}_a + A_{65}\ddot{\phi}_b + A_{66}\ddot{\phi}_c = B_6$$

All of the terms held in the coefficients A_{11} through B_6 can be derived from video or force data at each instant in time. A linear equation solver is used to determine estimates for the six unknowns at each time instant.

However, some of the equation coefficients involve $\cos\phi_a$, $\cos\phi_b$, $\cos\phi_c$ which result in singularities in the calculated torques and angular accelerations around $\phi_j = 90°$ ($j = a, b, c$). To avoid this problem a further three equations are added using video estimates e_1, e_2, e_3 of the angular accelerations $\ddot{\phi}_a, \ddot{\phi}_b, \ddot{\phi}_c$. These may be written as:

$$A_{44}\ddot{\phi}_a = A_{44}e_1$$
$$A_{55}\ddot{\phi}_b = A_{55}e_2$$
$$A_{66}\ddot{\phi}_c = A_{66}e_3$$

which match the coefficients of $\ddot{\phi}_a, \ddot{\phi}_b, \ddot{\phi}_c$ in the last three of the six previous equations. This gives an over-determined system of nine equations for the six unknowns and a least-squares equation solver results in solutions without singularities. The addition of the further three linear equations constrains the angular acceleration estimates returned by the solver to sensible values and consequently the torque values returned are also more stable (Figure 9.5).

In analysing movements with an impact phase, inverse dynamics is more problematic since it is not possible to include wobbling masses within an inverse

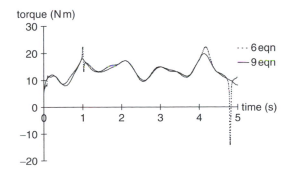

Figure 9.5 Joint torque obtained by inverse dynamics using six equation system and nine equation over-determined system. (Reproduced from Yeadon, M.R. and Trewartha, G. 2003. Control strategy for a hand balance. Motor Control 7, p. 418 by kind permission of Human Kinetics)

dynamics model. In such movements, a constrained forward dynamics model is a better way to proceed.

Solving the inverse dynamics problem using forwards dynamics simulation

An alternative to inverse dynamics is to use a constrained (angle-driven) forward dynamics simulation model for solving the inverse dynamics problem. This method allows wobbling masses to be included within the model, which can have a substantial effect on the joint torques calculated especially during impacts (Pain and Challis, 2006). The disadvantage of using a forward dynamics formulation is that it may be necessary to optimise model parameters to find a solution that matches the actual performance. In addition it is not possible to take advantage of an over-determined system and accurate acceleration values are needed, which can be almost impossible to calculate during impacts.

With a constrained forward dynamics planar model there are three degrees of freedom for whole body motion–horizontal and vertical translation of the mass centre and whole body orientation–along with three degrees of freedom for each wobbling mass segment in the model. Time histories of the joint angles and external forces are input to the model and the motion of the model is calculated along with the joint torques required to satisfy the joint angle changes. King *et al.*, 2003, used this method to calculate the net joint torque at the knee for the take-off phase in a jump for height. The peak knee torques calculated using quasi-static, pseudo-inverse dynamics (no wobbling mass movement), and constrained forward dynamics were 747 N m, 682 N m and 620 N m. Including segment accelerations resulted in lower peak values and the inclusion of wobbling masses resulted in a smoother knee torque time history. However, all the calculated peak knee torques were in excess of the eccentric maximum that could be exerted by the participant, which was estimated to be 277 N m from constant velocity experiments with the participant (Figure 9.6).

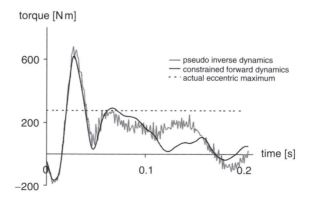

Figure 9.6 Knee joint torque calculated using pseudo inverse dynamics and constrained forward dynamics

King *et al.*, 2003, concluded that the discrepancy requires further investigation but it is likely to be due to modelling the knee as a simple frictionless pin joint or may be a consequence of errors in the digitised data.

APPLICATIONS

In this section various examples of modelling in sports biomechanics will be given, to illustrate model implementation and address the problems of optimisation and the control of sports movements.

Understanding the mechanics of sports technique

It is possible to use a simulation model to gain insight into the mechanics of sports techniques. Kinematic and kinetic data on an actual performance may suggest that a particular technique is responsible for the outcome but without some method of quantifying contributions little can be concluded. With a simulation model the efficacy of various techniques may be evaluated and so give insight into what really produces the resulting motion. Van Gheluwe, 1981, and Yeadon, 1993b; c, used angle-driven simulation models of aerial movement to investigate the capabilities of various contact and aerial twisting techniques. They found that twist could be produced in the aerial phase of a plain somersault using asymmetrical movements of arms or hips. Dapena, 1981, used an angle-driven model of the aerial phase of high jumping to show how a greater height could be cleared by modifying the configuration changes during flight.

Simulation models have provided insight into the mechanics of technique in: the flight phase of springboard diving (Miller, 1971), circling a high bar (Arampatz and Brüggemann., 1999; Arampatzis *et al.*, 2001; Hiley and Yeadon, 2001), skateboarding (Hubbard, 1980), the curved approach in high jumping (Tan, 1997), and landings in gymnastics (Requejo *et al.*, 2004). It is important, however, that a model is evaluated before it is applied, since the insights gained may be into the, possibly incorrect, model rather than into actual performance.

Contributions

Simulation models may be used to determine the contributions of various aspects to the overall performance by simulating the effect of what happens when an aspect is removed or when just one aspect is present. So that a variable can be used to quantify 'contributions' it is necessary that such measures are additive. For example, in twisting somersaults the use of the final twist angle achieved can lead to problems since the sum of twist angles produced by various techniques is likely to be greater than the twist resulting from the concurrent use of all the techniques. Additionally, technique in the latter part of a twisting somersault may be primarily directed towards stopping the twist rather than producing the twist. Because of these effects Yeadon, 1993d, used the maximum tilt angle as a measure of the twist potential in a movement. The tilt angles calculated in this way were additive and could be sensibly referred to as contributions from various twisting techniques.

Brewin et al., 2000, used a model of a gymnast and the rings apparatus to determine the contributions of technique and the elasticity of the gymnast and rings apparatus to the reduction of loading at the shoulders. It was found that technique reduced the loading by 2.7 body weights while elasticity reduced the loading by 1.1 body weights resulting in the actual loading of 8.5 body weights. King and Yeadon, 2005, used a five-segment model of a gymnast during vaulting take-off to investigate factors affecting performance of the Hecht vault. It was found that shoulder torque made only a small contribution of 7° to the resulting rotation whereas shoulder elasticity contributed 50° to the rotation in flight.

Optimisation of sports technique

Since a single simulation of a sports movement might take around one second it is possible to run thousands of simulations in a single day. This opens the way to investigating optimised performance by means of a theoretical study. The technique used in a sports movement is characterised using various parameters and then an optimisation procedure is used to find the best set of parameter values that maximises or minimises some performance score.

At its simplest, this could involve determining the optimal initial conditions in a projectile event such as basketball (Schwark et al., 2004) or javelin (Best et al., 1995; Hubbard and Alaways, 1987). Similarly, optimum bat swing trajectories can be determined for maximum baseball range (Sawicki et al., 2003). In such optimisations relatively few parameters corresponding to one instant in time are optimised. In such cases it is important to take account of the inter-dependence of release parameters arising from the characteristics of the human participant (Hubbard et al., 2001).

More challenging are dynamic optimisations in which the time history of a sports technique is optimised. Typically this requires many parameters to characterise the technique used. In the case of angle-driven models, it is relatively simple to ensure that anatomical constraints at the joints are not violated (Hiley and Yeadon, 2003a). For models driven by joint torques or muscle representations, such constraints cannot be imposed directly but can be accommodated using penalties as part of the optimisation function (Kong et al., 2005).

The performance score of the sports skill could simply be the distance thrown (Hubbard, 1984) or the distance jumped (Hatze, 1983; Hubbard et al., 1989), the height jumped (Nagano and Gerritsen, 2001; Cheng and Hubbard, 2004), the amount of rotation produced (Sprigings and Miller, 2004; Hiley and Yeadon, 2005), power output (van den Bogert, 1994), fatigue (Neptune and Hull, 1999) or more complex combinations of performance variables (Gervais, 1994; Koh et al., 2003). While such an approach may work it is also possible that the optimum solution is sensitive to small variations in technique, leading to inconsistent performance. This issue of robustness to perturbations will be discussed in the next section.

CONTROL OF SPORTS MOVEMENTS

If a technique produces a perfect performance then inevitably there will be deviations from this performance resulting from small errors in timing. If the magnitude of such timing errors is known then the performance error can be calculated or, conversely, the timing errors may be estimated from the performance error. Yeadon and Brewin, 2003, estimated that timing errors were of the order of 15 ms for a longswing to a still handstand on rings.

Some movements, such as a hand balance on floor (Yeadon and Trewartha, 2003) or a non-twisting straight somersault (Yeadon and Mikulcik, 1996), may be inherently unstable and may require continual proprioceptive feedback control to be performed at all. Other movements, such as twisting somersaults (Yeadon, 2001; 2002), may require continual feedback correction to prevent drift away from the targeted performance. Variation in approach characteristics in tumbling may be compensated for by modifications in take-off technique using feed-forward control but only if such variation can be estimated in advance with sufficient accuracy (King and Yeadon, 2003).

Variation in technique can also be coped with by adopting a technique that is relatively insensitive, or robust, to perturbations (van Soest *et al.*, 1994; King and Yeadon, 2004). In cases where the limits of timing a movement are close to being reached, such considerations may be the main driver for selecting technique (Hiley and Yeadon, 2003b).

CONDUCTING A STUDY

The main steps in conducting a study using a simulation model are as follows:

- identification of the research questions to be addressed
- design of the model with these aims in mind
- model construction
- data collection for model input and parameter determination
- parameter determination
- model evaluation
- experimental design of simulations to be run
- results of simulations
- conclusions: answering the research questions.

REPORTING A STUDY

The format for reporting on a study will depend to some extent on the intended readership but should reflect the main steps listed in the previous section. Figures should be used when presenting a description of the model, performance data, simulation output, and model evaluation comparisons. The structure of a report or paper is usually along the following traditional lines:

- introduction: background, statement of aims
- methods: model design, parameter determination, data collection, evaluation
- results: simulation output, graphs, graphics, tables
- discussion: addressing the aims, limitations, conclusions.

SUMMARY

The use of simulation models in sport can give insight into what is happening or, in the case of a failing model, what is not happening (Niklas, 1992). Models also provide a means for testing hypotheses generated from observations or measurements of performance. It should be remembered, however, that all models are simplifications and will not reflect all aspects of the real system. The strength of computer simulation modelling in providing sports science support for performers is that it can provide general research results for the understanding of elite performance. While there is also the possibility of providing individual advice using personalised models, most sports biomechanics practitioners are a long way from realising this at present.

REFERENCES

Alexander, R.M. (1990) 'Optimum take-off techniques for high and long jumps', *Philosophical Transactions of the Royal Society of London – Series B*: 329: 3–10.

Alexander, R.M. (2003) 'Modelling approaches in biomechanics', *Philosophical Transactions of the Royal Society of London – Series B: Biological Sciences*, 358: 1429–1435.

Arampatzis, A. and Brüggemann, G.-P. (1999) 'Mechanical energetic processes during the giant swing exercise before dismounts and flight elements on the high bar and the uneven parallel bars', *Journal of Biomechanics*, 32: 811–820.

Arampatzis, A., Brüggemann, G.-P. and Klapsing, G.M. (2001) 'Mechanical energetic processes during the giant swing before the Tkatchev exercise', *Journal of Biomechanics*, 34: 505–512.

Best, R.J., Bartlett, R.M. and Sawyer, R.A. (1995) 'Optimal javelin release', *Journal of Applied Biomechanics*, 11: 371–394.

Bobbert, M.F., Houdijk, J.H.P., Koning, J.J. de and Groot, G. de (2002) 'From a one-Legged vertical jump to the speed-skating push-off: A simulation study', *Journal of Applied Biomechanics*, 18: 28–45.

Brewin, M.A., Yeadon, M.R. and Kerwin, D.G. (2000) 'Minimising peak forces at the shoulders during backward longswings on rings', *Human Movement Science*, 19: 717–736.

Caldwell, G.E. (2004) 'Muscle modeling', in G.E. Robertson, G.E. Caldwell, J. Hamill, G. Kamen, S.N. and Whittlesey (eds), *Research Methods in Biomechanics*, Champaign, IL: Human Kinetics.

Chandler, R.F., Clauser, C.E., McConville, J.T., Reynolds, H.M. and Young, J.W. (1975) 'Investigation of inertial properties of the human body. *AMRL T R* 74–137, AD-A016-485, DOT-HS-801-430. Wright-Patterson Air Force Base, Ohio.

Chapman, A.E. (1985) 'The mechanical properties of human muscle', in R.L. Terjung (ed.) *Exercise and Sport Sciences Reviews–Volume 13*, London: MacMillan.

Cheng, K.B. and Hubbard, M. (2004) 'Optimal jumping strategies from compliant surfaces: A simple model of springboard standing jumps', *Human Movement Science*, 23: 35–48.

Clarys, J.P. and Marfell-Jones, M.J. (1986) 'Anthropometric prediction of component tissue masses in the minor limb segments of the human body', *Human Biology*, 58: 761–769.

Dapena, J. (1981) 'Simulation of modified human airborne movements', *Journal of Biomechanics*, 14: 81–89.

Dempster, W.T. (1955) 'Space requirements of the seated operator', *Wright Air Development Centre*, Wight-Paterson Air Force Base, Ohio WADC-TR: 55–159.

De Zee, M. and Voigt, M. (2001) 'Moment dependency of the series elastic stiffness in the human plantar flexors measured in vivo', *Journal of Biomechanics*, 34: 1399–1406.

Dudley, G.A., Harris, R.T., Duvoisin, M.R., Hather, B.M. and Buchanan, P. (1990) 'Effect of voluntary vs. artificial activation on the relationship of muscle torque to speed', *Journal of Applied Physiology*, 69: 2215–2221.

Edman, K.A.P. (1992) 'Contractile performance of skeletal muscle fibres', in P.V. Komi (ed.), *Strength and Power in Sport. Vol. III of the Encyclopaedia of Sports Medicine*, Oxford: Blackwell Scientific.

Fujii, N. and Hubbard, M. (2002) 'Validation of a three-dimensional baseball pitching model', *Journal of Applied Biomechanics*, 18: 135–154.

Gerritsen, K.G.M., van den Bogert, A.J. and Nigg, B.M. (1995) 'Direct dynamics simulation of the impact phase in heel–toe running', *Journal of Biomechanics*, 28: 661–68.

Gervais, P. (1994) 'A prediction of an optimal performance of the handspring 1½ front salto longhorse vault', *Journal of Biomechanics*, 27: 67–75.

Greig, M.P. and Yeadon, M.R. (2000) 'The influence of touchdown parameters on the performance of a high jumper', *Journal of Applied Biomechanics*, 16: 367–378.

Gruber, K., Ruder, H., Denoth, J. and Schneider, K. (1998) 'A comparative study of impact dynamics: wobbling mass model versus rigid body models', *Journal of Biomechanics*, 31: 439–444.

Goffe, W.L., Ferrier, G.D. and Rogers, J. (1994) 'Global optimisation of statistical functions with simulated annealing', *Journal of Econometrics*, 60: 65–99.

Harry, J.D., Ward, A.W., Heglund, N.C., Morgan, D.L. and McMahon, T.A. (1990) 'Cross-bridge cycling theories cannot explain high-speed lengthening behaviour in frog muscle', *Biophysical Journal*, 57: 201–208.

Hatze, H. (1980) 'A mathematical model for the computational determination of parameter values of anthropomorphic segments', *Journal of Biomechanics*, 13: 833–843.

Hatze, H. (1981a) 'A comprehensive model for human motion simulation and its application to the take-off phase of the long jump', *Journal of Biomechanics*, 14: 135–142.

Hatze, H. (1981b) 'Estimation of myodynamic parameter values from observations on isometrically contracting muscle groups', *European Journal of Applied Physiology*, 46: 325–338.

Hatze, H. (1983) 'Computerized optimization of sports motions: An overview of possibilities, methods and recent developments', *Journal of Sports Sciences*, 1: 3–12.

Hiley, M.J. and Yeadon, M.R. (2001) 'Swinging around the high bar', *Physics Education*, 36, 1: 14–17.

Hiley, M.J. and Yeadon, M.R. (2003a) 'Optimum technique for generating angular momentum in accelerated backward giant circles prior to a dismount', *Journal of Applied Biomechanics*, 19: 119–130.

Hiley, M.J. and Yeadon, M.R. (2003b) 'The margin for error when releasing the high bar for dismounts', *Journal of Biomechanics*, 36: 313–319.

Hiley, M.J. and Yeadon, M.R. (2005) 'Maximal dismounts from high bar', *Journal of Biomechanics*, 38: 2221–2227.

Hill, A.V. (1938) 'The heat of shortening and the dynamic constants of muscle', *Proceedings of the Royal Society Series B*, 126: 136–195.

Hinrichs, R.N. (1985) 'Regression equations to predict segmental moments of inertia from anthropometric measurements: An extension of the data of Chandler *et al.* (1975)', *Journal of Biomechanics*, 18: 621–624.

Hubbard, M. (1980) 'Human control of the skateboard', *Journal of Biomechanics*, 13: 745–754.

Hubbard, M. (1984) 'Optimal javelin trajectories', *Journal of Biomechanics*, 17: 777–787.

Hubbard, M. (1993) 'Computer Simulation in Sport and Industry', *Journal of Biomechanics*, 26, Supplement 1: 53–61.

Hubbard, M. and Trinkle, J.C. (1985a) 'Clearing maximum height with constrained kinetic energy', *ASME Journal of Applied Mechanics*, 52: 179–184.

Hubbard, M. and Trinkle, J.C. (1985b) 'Optimal Fosbury-flop high jumping', in D.A. Winter, R.W. Norman, R.P. Wells, K.C. Hayes and A.E. Patla (eds), *Biomechanics IX-B*, Champaign, IL: Human Kinetics.

Hubbard, M. and Alaways, L.W. (1987) 'Optimum release conditions for the new rules javelin', *International Journal of Sport Biomechanics*, 3: 207–221.

Hubbard, M. and Alaways, L.W. (1989) 'Rapid and accurate estimation of release conditions in the javelin throw', *Journal of Biomechanics*, 22: 583–596.

Hubbard, M., Hibbard, R.L., Yeadon, M.R. and Komor, A. (1989) 'A multisegment dynamic model of ski jumping', *International Journal of Sport Biomechanics*, 5: 258–274.

Hubbard, M., de Mestre, N.J. and Scott, J. (2001) 'Dependence of release variables in the shot put', *Journal of Biomechanics*, 34: 449–456.

Jensen, R.K. (1978) 'Estimation of the biomechanical properties of three body types using a photogrammetric method', *Journal of Biomechanics*, 11: 349–358.

King, A.I. (1984) 'A review of biomechanical models', *Journal of Biomechanical Engineering*, 106: 97–104.

King, M.A. and Yeadon, M.R. (2002) 'Determining subject specific torque parameters for use in a torque driven simulation model of dynamic jumping', *Journal of Applied Biomechanics*, 18: 207–217.

King, M.A. and Yeadon, M.R. (2003) 'Coping with perturbations to a layout somersault in tumbling', *Journal of Biomechanics*, 36: 921–927.

King, M.A. and Yeadon, M.R. (2004) 'Maximising somersault rotation in tumbling', *Journal of Biomechanics*, 37: 471–477.

King, M.A. and Yeadon, M.R. (2005) 'Factors influencing performance in the Hecht vault and implications for modelling', *Journal of Biomechanics*, 38: 145–151.

King, M.A., Yeadon, M.R. and Kerwin, D.G. (1999) 'A two segment simulation model of long horse vaulting', *Journal of Sports Sciences*, 17: 313–324.

King, M.A., Wilson, C. and Yeadon, M.R. (2003) 'Determination of knee joint moments during running jumps using a constrained forward dynamics simulation model', *International Journal of Computer Science in Sport*, 2: 102–103.

King, M.A., Wilson, C. and Yeadon, M.R. (2006) 'Evaluation of a torque-driven computer simulation model of jumping for height', *Journal of Applied Biomechanics*, 22: 264–274.

Koh, M., Jennings, L., Elliott, B. and Lloyd, D. (2003) 'A predicted optimal performance of the Yurchenko layout vault in women's artistic gymnastics', *Journal of Applied Biomechanics*, 19: 187–204.

Kong, P.W., Yeadon, M.R. and King, M.A. (2005) 'Optimisation of take-off techniques for maximum forward rotation in springboard diving', in Q. Wang (ed.) *XXIII International Symposium on Biomechanics in Sports*, Beijing: The China Institute of Sport Science.

Martin, P.E., Mungiole, M., Marzke, M.W. and Longhill, J.M. (1989) 'The use of magnetic resonance imaging for measuring segment inertial properties', *Journal of Biomechanics*, 22: 367–369.

Miller, D.I. (1971) 'A computer simulation of the airborne phase of diving', in J.M. Cooper (ed.), *Selected Topics on Biomechanics*, Chicago, IL: Athletic Institute.

Miller, D.I. (1975) 'Computer simulation of human motion', in D.W Grieve, D.I. Miller, D. Mitchelson, J. Paul and A.J. Smith (eds), *Techniques for the Analysis of Human Movement*, London: Lepus Books.

Muramatsu, T., Muraoka, T., Takeshita, D., Kawakami, Y., Hirano, Y. and Fukunaga, T. (2001) 'Mechanical properties of tendon and aponeurosis of human gastrocnemius muscle in vivo', *Journal of Applied Physiology*, 90: 1671–1678.

Nagano, A. and Gerritsen, G.M. (2001) 'Effects of neuromuscular strength training on vertical jumping performance – A computer simulation study', *Journal of Applied Biomechanics*, 17: 113–128.

Nelder, J.A. and Mead, R. (1965) 'A simplex method for function minimisation', *Computer Journal*, 7: 308–313.

Neptune, R.R. and Hull, M.L. (1998) 'Evaluation of performance criteria for simulation of submaximal steady-state cycling using a forward dynamic model', *Journal of Biomechanical Engineering*, 120: 334–341.

Neptune, R.R. and Hull, M.L. (1999) 'A theoretical analysis of preferred pedaling rate selection in endurance cycling', *Journal of Biomechanics*, 32: 409–415.

Neptune, R.R. and Kautz, S.A. (2000) 'Knee joint loading in forward versus backward pedaling: implications for rehabilitation strategies', *Clinical Biomechanics*, 15: 528–535.

Niklas, K.J. (1992) *Plant Biomechanics: an Engineering Approach to Plant Form and Function*, Chicago, IL: University of Chicago Press.

Pain, M.T.G. and Challis, J.H. (2001a) 'High resolution determination of body segment inertial parameters and their variation due to soft tissue motion', *Journal of Applied Biomechanics*, 17: 326–334.

Pain, M.T.G. and Challis, J.H. (2001b) 'The role of the heel pad and shank soft tissue during impacts: a further resolution of a paradox', *Journal of Biomechanics*, 34: 327–333.

Pain, M.T.G. and Challis, J.H. (2006) 'The influence of soft tissue movement on ground reaction forces, joint torques and joint reaction forces in drop landings', *Journal of Biomechanics*, 39: 119–124.

Panjabi, M. (1979) 'Validation of mathematical models', *Journal of Biomechanics*, 12: 238.

Press, W.H., Flannery, B.P., Teukolsky, S.A. and Vetterling, W.T. (1988) *Numerical Recipes. The Art of Scientific Computing*, Cambridge: Cambridge University Press.

Requejo, P.S., McNitt-Gray, J.L. and Flashner, H. (2004) 'Modification of landing conditions at contact via flight phase control', *Biological Cybernetics*, 90: 327–336.

Sawicki, G.S., Hubbard, M. and Stronge, W.J. (2003) 'How to hit home runs: Optimum baseball bat swing parameters for maximum range trajectories', *American Journal of Physics*, 71: 1152–1162.

Schwark, B.N., Mackenzie, S.J. and Sprigings, E.J. (2004) 'Optimizing the release conditions for a free throw in wheelchair basketball', *Journal of Applied Biomechanics*, 20: 153–166.

Sprigings, E.J. and Yeadon, M.R. (1997) 'An insight into the reversal of rotation in the Hecht vault', *Human Movement Science*, 16: 517–532.

Sprigings, E.J. and Miller, D.I. (2004) 'Optimal knee extension timing in springboard and platform dives from the reverse group', *Journal of Applied Biomechanics*, 20: 244–252.

Sprigings, E.J., Lanovaz, J.L., Watson, L.G. and Russell, K.W. (1998) 'Removing swing from a handstand on rings using a properly timed backward giant circle: a simulation solution', *Journal of Biomechanics*, 31: 27–35.

Tan, J.C.C. (1997) 'The mechanics of the curved approach in high jumping' Unpublished doctoral dissertation, Loughborough University, UK.

Van den Bogert, A.J. (1994) 'Optimization of the human engine: application to sprint cycling', in W. Herzog, B. Nigg and T. van den Bogert (eds), *Canadian Society for Biomechanics: Proceedings of the Eight Biennial Conference and Symposium*, Calgary: Canadian Society for Biomechanics.

Van der Helm, F.C.T. (1994) 'A finite element musculoskeletal model of the shoulder mechanism', *Journal of Biomechanics*, 27: 551–569.

Van Gheluwe, B. (1981) 'A biomechanical simulation model for airborne twist in backward somersault', *Journal of Human Movement Studies*, 7: 1–22.

Van Soest, A.J., Bobbert, M.F. and Ingen Schenau, G.J. van (1994) 'A control strategy for the execution of explosive movements from varying starting positions', *Journal of Neurophysiology*, 71: 1390–1402.

Van Soest A.J. and Casius, L.J.R. (2003) 'The merits of a parallel genetic algorithm in solving hard optimization problems', *Journal of Biomechanical Engineering*, 125: 141–146.

Vaughan, C.L. (1984) 'Computer simulation of human motion in sports biomechanics', in R.L. Terjung (ed.), *Exercise and Sport Sciences Reviews – Volume 12*, New York: MacMillan.

Vaughan, C.L. (ed.) (1989) *Biomechanics of Sport*, Boca Raton, FL: CRC Press.

Westing, S.H., Seger, J.Y., Karlson, E. and Ekblom, B. (1988) 'Eccentric and concentric torque-velocity characteristics of the quadriceps femoris in man', *European Journal of Applied Physiology*, 58: 100–104.

Wilson, C., King, M.A. and Yeadon, M.R. (2006) 'Determination of subject-specific model parameter visco-elastic elements', *Journal of Biomechanics*, 39: 1883–1890.

Wright, I.C., Neptune, R.R., van den Bogert, A.J. and Nigg, B.M. (1998) 'Passive regulation of impact forces in heel–toe running', *Clinical Biomechanics*, 13: 521–531.

Yeadon, M.R. (1987) 'Theoretical models and their application to aerial movement', in J. Atha and B. van Gheluwe (eds), *Medicine and Sport Science, 25: Current Research in Sports Biomechanics*, Basel: Karger.

Yeadon, M.R. (1990a) 'The simulation of aerial movement–I: The determination of orientation angles from film data', *Journal of Biomechanics*, 23: 59–66.

Yeadon, M.R. (1990b) 'The simulation of aerial movement–II: A mathematical inertia model of the human body', *Journal of Biomechanics*, 23: 67–74.

Yeadon, M.R. (1993a) 'The biomechanics of twisting somersaults. Part I: Rigid body motions', *Journal of Sports Sciences*, 11: 187-198.

Yeadon, M.R. (1993b) 'The biomechanics of twisting somersaults. Part II: Contact twist', *Journal of Sports Sciences*, 11: 199–208.

Yeadon, M.R. (1993c) 'The biomechanics of twisting somersaults. Part III: Aerial twist', *Journal of Sports Sciences*, 11: 209–218.

Yeadon, M.R. (1993d) 'The biomechanics of twisting somersaults. Part IV: Partitioning performance using the tilt angle', *Journal of Sports Sciences*, 11: 219–225.

Yeadon, M.R. (2001) The control of twisting somersaults, in R. Mueller, H. Gerber and A. Stacoff (eds), *XVIIIth Congress of the International Society of Biomechanics, Book of Abstracts*, Zurich: ETH.

Yeadon, M.R. (2002) 'The control of twisting somersaults using asymmetrical arm movements', in *IV World Congress of Biomechanics Proceedings CD*, University of Calgary, Calgary, Canada.

Yeadon, M.R. and Morlock, M. (1989) 'The appropriate use of regression equations for the estimation of segmental inertia parameters', *Journal of Biomechanics*, 22: 683–689.

Yeadon, M.R. and Challis, J.H. (1994) 'The future of performance related sports biomechanics research', *Journal of Sports Sciences*, 12: 3–32.

Yeadon, M.R. and Mikulcik, E.C. (1996) 'The control of non-twisting somersaults using configurational changes', *Journal of Biomechanics*, 29: 1341–1348.

Yeadon, M.R. and Hiley, M.J. (2000) 'The mechanics of the backward giant circle on the high bar', *Human Movement Science*, 19: 153–173.

Yeadon, M.R. and King, M.A. (2002) 'Evaluation of a torque driven simulation model of tumbling', *Journal of Applied Biomechanics*, 18: 195–206.

Yeadon, M.R. and Brewin, M.A. (2003) 'Optimised performance of the backward longswing on rings', *Journal of Biomechanics*, 36: 545–552.

Yeadon, M.R. and Trewartha, G. (2003) 'Control strategy for a hand balance', *Motor Control*, 7: 411–430.

Yeadon, M.R., Atha, J. and Hales, F.D. (1990) 'The simulation of aerial movement–IV: A computer simulation model', *Journal of Biomechanics*, 23: 85–89.

Yeadon, M.R., King, M.A. and Wilson, C. (2006a) 'Modelling the maximum voluntary joint torque/angular velocity relationship in human movement', *Journal of Biomechanics*, 39: 476–482.

Yeadon, M.R., Kong, P.W. and King, M.A. (2006b) 'Parameter determination for a computer simulation model of a diver and a springboard', *Journal of Applied Biomechanics*, 22: 167–176.

Zatsiorsky, V.M. (2002) *Kinetics of Human Motion*, Champaign, IL: Human Kinetics.

Zatsiorsky, V.M., Seluyanov, V.N. and Chugunova, L. (1990) 'In vivo body segment inertial parameters determination using a gamma-scanner method', in N. Berme and A. Cappozzo (eds), *Biomechanics of Human Movement: Applications in Rehabilitation, Sports and Ergonomics*, Worthington, OH: Bertec Corporation.

THE BRITISH ASSOCIATION OF SPORT AND EXERCISE SCIENCES–CODE OF CONDUCT

INTRODUCTION

This code of conduct sets out the principles of conduct and ethics for the guidance of members of the British Association of Sport and Exercise Sciences (BASES) and its three constituent Divisions: Education and Professional Development; Physical Activity for Health; and Sport and Performance. All members of BASES are bound by the provisions of this code of conduct and each Division's own professional guidelines, which provide further detail in respect of experimental techniques, protocols and analysis procedures, the obtaining of medico-legal clearance and informed consent. BASES members are reminded that the aims of the Association are:

(a) the promotion of research in sport and exercise sciences
(b) the encouragement of evidence-based practice in sport and exercise sciences
(c) the distribution of knowledge in sport and exercise sciences
(d) the development and maintenance of high professional standards for those involved in sport and exercise sciences
(e) the representation of the interests of sport and exercise sciences nationally and internationally.

Throughout this Code of Conduct the word 'client(s)' includes all participants. In both, carrying out these aims and their working practices, BASES members must take into account the three following principles:

(a) all clients have the right to expect the highest standards of professionalism, consideration and respect
(b) the pursuit of scientific knowledge requires that research and testing is carried out with utmost integrity

(c)   the law requires that working practices are safe and that the welfare of the client is paramount.

STRUCTURE

Members are reminded that the authority of BASES is vested in the Strategic Management Team, which alone has the power to review and recommend amendment to this code of conduct. Any questions arising from this code of conduct or its interpretation (apart from disciplinary matters for which see section 9) shall be referred at first by any member to the Strategic Management Team for final determination. Any member aggrieved by the decision of a Division Chair may appeal to the Strategic Management Team for a ruling, whose decision shall be final.

ETHICAL CLEARANCE

Ethical clearance must be obtained from an appropriate Local Ethics Committee or similar local body for non-routine work undertaken by members. Specific clearance must always be obtained before the imposition of any unusual or severe physical or psychological stress, the administration of any ergogenic aid, working with clients with disabilities, or the employment of biopsy or venipuncture. The list is not exhaustive and specific clearance is often required in other areas of work, such as with children, vunerable adults or the sampling of capillary blood. If any members is in doubt as to whether ethical clearance is required, an assessment of risk should be carried out and if there is any remaining doubt reference should be made, in advance, to the local ethics committee or body.

INFORMED CONSENT AND CONFIDENTIALITY

(a)   Informed consent

No member may undertake any work without first having the informed consent of all participating clients. Informed consent is the knowing consent of a client (or legally authorised representative in the case of the child) who is in a position to exercise free power of choice without any undue inducement or element of force, fraud, deceit or coercion.

In most cases, informed consent may be obtained by having the client read and sign a document setting out all of the information relevant to the proposed investigation or test. This would normally included a description of the investigation and its objectives, the procedures to be followed, an outline of the risks and benefits, an offer to answer any queries, an instruction that the client is free to withdraw at any point without prejudice, together with an explanation concerning confidentiality.

In some cases (e.g. simple field tests), informed consent may be obtained verbally but in every such case members must make an appropriate written record confirming that informed consent had been obtained. Where a full explanation to a client may adversely affect the work, members must obtain prior local ethics committee consent to provide a more general outline of the aims of the investigation and the committee may set out the extent of the information to be given at its discretion.

(b)   Confidentiality

It is of paramount importance that all BASES members must preserve the confidentiality of the information acquired in their work which must not be devolved with out prior written consent of a client. All clients must be informed that they have a right to a copy of such information relating the them and all members must supply a copy if so requested. It is deemed to be good practice to supply copies in any event, as a matter of course.

DATA PROTECTION AND RESPONSIBILITY

(a)   Storage and use of individually identifiable data must be in accordance with the provisions of the Data Protection Act 1998.

(b)   The obtaining of data and its presentation/publication must be unbiased and responsible. Validity, objectivity and reliability are key principles and caution should be exercised with the interpretation and explanation of test results.

(c)   Members should seek to maximise the accessibility of research findings and, wherever appropriate, publish them in the interest of both science, and sport and exercise.

(d)   Publication of data must not disclose the identity of any individual client unless the prior written consent of the individual is obtained.

COMPETENCE

(a)   Members must recognise their limitations in qualifications, experience, expertise and competence and must operate within these limits, restricting the interpretation of results to those, which they are qualified to give and in employing any equipment and techniques, which they are qualified to use.

(b)   Any matter, whose essence appears to lie within another specialist field such as medicine or physiotherapy, or another discipline within BASES, must be referred to an appropriate professional within such a field.

(c)   Members must not misrepresent their qualifications, experience or expertise in any way or exaggerate or mislead clients in respect of the effectiveness of any techniques they undertake.

(d)   Professional members should seek to become accredited where and when appropriate.

(e)   All members must be knowledgeable in respect of contemporary research and practice.

PROFESSIONAL AND PERSONAL CONDUCT

(a)   Members' paramount concern is the well-being of their clients.

(b)   Members must conduct themselves in such a way that brings credit to their specialist areas.

(c)   Members must not practise or work when they are not fit to operate effectively and professionally.

(d)   Members must not exploit relationships with clients for personal gain or gratification.

(e)   Members must not in any way jeopardise the safety or interests of clients.

(f)   Members must be totally unbiased and objective in their practices and actions.

(g)   Members must ensure, where appropriate, the highest standards of safety and working practices and research both in respect of work undertaken by members themselves or by others under their supervision.

(h)   Members must respond, with all due expedition, to any enquiry from any client or any other member of BASES or any committee of BASES.

(i)   Members must ensure that suitable insurance indemnity cover is in place for all areas of work that they undertake.

(j)   Members must not do any act or thing, or omit to do any act or thing which in any way brings, or is likely to bring, BASES into disrepute.

OFFICERS

All officers of BASES and the individual Divisions must:

(a)   act with strict impartiality with respect of any matter referred to them for consideration as officers,

(b)   use their best endeavours to make the best use of all resources available to BASES in the interests of BASES and its members,

(c)   make a prior declaration in respect of any matter in which they have direct or indirect personal interest,

(d)   not take part in any part of or vote on any matter in which they have a direct or indirect personal interest.

DISCIPLINARY PROCEDURES

(a) Any person (whether or not a member) may make a complaint that a member has failed to comply with this code of conduct. Members are under an obligation to report all instances of breaches of this code.

(b) Such complaint shall be made in writing to the Honorary Secretary of BASES.

(c) Upon receiving a complaint, the Honorary Secretary must investigate it is soon as possible unless the complaint is anonymous in which case the Secretary has the discretion as to whether to investigate it or not. The Honorary Secretary shall investigate any complaint impartially and with the assistance of a salaried member of the BASES staff or other nominated officer.

(d) The member shall receive full written details of the complaint against them.

(e) The member shall respond in writing within 28 days of receiving details of the complaint.

(f) The Honorary Secretary shall cause all such relevant enquiries to be made as the Honorary Secretary considers necessary to ascertain the validity or otherwise of the complaint and, as soon as possible thereafter, the Honorary Secretary shall refer the matter to a disciplinary tribunal.

(g) The disciplinary tribunal shall comprise the Chair of BASES, Division Chair of the member's Division and one other Division Chair and a BASES legal representative if deemed necessary.

(h) The disciplinary tribunal shall meet as soon as conveniently possible to consider the complaint and will give reasonable notice to the member of the time, date and place of disciplinary tribunals meeting.

(i) The member shall be entitle to attend the tribunal in person (with a representative if they so wish who must be identified 14 days before the tribunal meets) and shall be entitled to a copy of all documentation that the tribunal is considering.

(j) The tribunal may call any person to give information to it and the member shall be entitled to ask any relevant questions of such person and shall be entitled to address the tribunal. Subject to this, the disciplinary tribunal shall have the power to decide the form and nature of any hearing but any such procedure must be fair and reasonable to all parties.

(k) At the conclusion of the hearing, the disciplinary tribunal must adjudicate on the complaint and decision may reached by a majority.

(l) In the event that the complaint is upheld the disciplinary tribunal shall have full discretion to impose any of the following penalties on any member:

   (i)   a written caution as to future behaviour
   (ii) a fine
   (iii) suspension from membership for a fixed period
   (iv) expulsion from membership

(m) Prior to the imposition of suspension or expulsion a member must be provided with the opportunity to make a written or personal presentation to the tribunal.

(n) Written notice of any penalty imposed shall be given to the member and a copy may be circulated to any other member.

(o) On being presented with any new relevant evidence the tribunal has the discretionary power to review any complaint and may, on any such review, review not only its prior decision but also any penalty imposed whether by reducing, increasing or cancelling the same.

(p) If any member is aggrieved by the decision of the disciplinary tribunal, he or she may, within fourteen days of receiving the written decision of the disciplinary tribunal, appeal the decision to the Strategic Management Team who shall have full power to consider the matter afresh, excluding the original tribunal member, together with full power to reduce, increase, cancel or confirm any penalty imposed.

21 February 2006
Copyright © BASES, 2006

ON-LINE MOTION ANALYSIS SYSTEM MANUFACTURERS AND THEIR WEBSITES

Charnwood Dynamics	www.charndyn.com
Elite Biomechanics	www.bts.it
Motion Analysis Corporation	www.motionanalysis.com
Northern Digital Inc.	www.ndigital.com
Peak Performance Technologies	www.peakperform.com
Qualisys Medical AB	www.qualisys.com
Skill Technologies Inc.	www.skilltechnologies.com
Vicon Motion Systems	www.vicon.com

INDEX

DATE DUE
